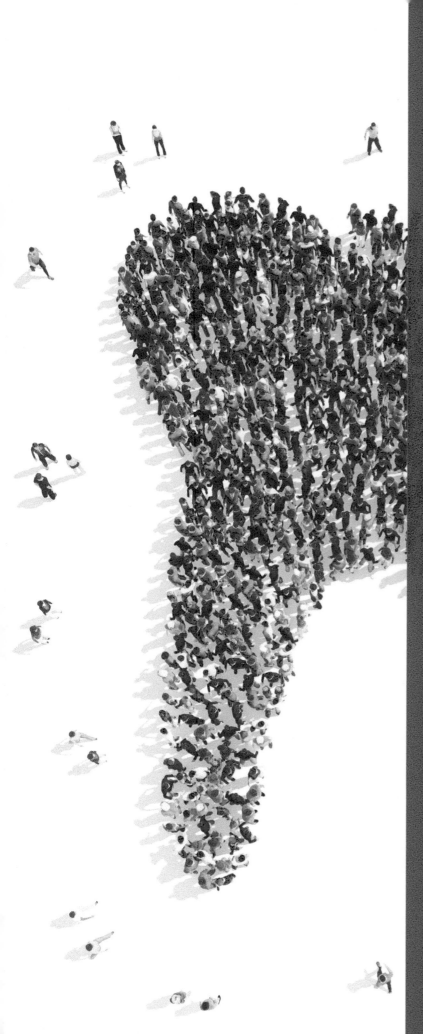

Dental Public Health

at a Glance

Second Edition

Ivor G. Chestnutt

BDS, MPH, PhD, FDS (DPH) RCSEdin, DDPH,
FDS RCSEng, FDS RCPSGlas, FFPH, FHEA
Professor and Honorary Consultant in Dental
Public Health
School of Dentistry
Cardiff University
Cardiff
UK

WILEY Blackwell

Registered Office
John Wiley & Sons, Inc., 111 River Street, Hoboken, NJ 07030, USA
John Wiley & Sons Ltd, The Atrium, Southern Gate, Chichester, West Sussex, PO19 8SQ, UK

For details of our global editorial offices, customer services, and more information about Wiley products visit us at www.wiley.com.

Wiley also publishes its books in a variety of electronic formats and by print-on-demand. Some content that appears in standard print versions of this book may not be available in other formats.

Library of Congress Cataloging-in-Publication Data

Names: Chestnutt, I. G., author.
Title: Dental public health at a glance / Ivor G. Chestnutt.
Description: Second edition. | Hoboken, NJ : Wiley, 2024. | Includes
    bibliographical references and index.
Identifiers: LCCN 2024000381 (print) | LCCN 2024000382 (ebook) | ISBN
    9781394184316 (paperback) | ISBN 9781394184286 (adobe pdf) | ISBN
    9781394184309 (epub)
Subjects: MESH: Public Health Dentistry | Dental Health Services | Oral
    Health | Handbook
Classification: LCC RK52 (print) | LCC RK52 (ebook) | NLM WU 49 | DDC
    362.1976–dc23/eng/20240207
LC record available at https://lccn.loc.gov/2024000381
LC ebook record available at https://lccn.loc.gov/2024000382

Cover Design: Wiley
Cover Image: © tai11/Shutterstock

Set in 9.5/11.5pt Minion Pro by Straive, Pondicherry, India
SKY10075634_052224

Contents

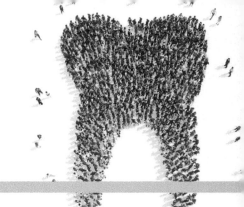

Preface from the first edition

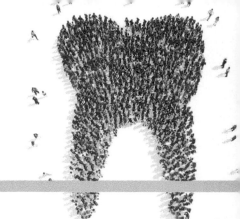

Members of the dental team are in a unique position to offer tailored and personalised advice and to thereby educate their patients on the steps that are necessary to secure oral health. However, there is only so much that can be achieved by such one-to-one, 'downstream' interventions. It is crucial that all members of the dental team appreciate the wider determinants of health and the impact of lifestyle and life circumstances on the health and oral health of their patients. The population has not benefited equally from the significant improvements in oral health observed over the past four decades. That one-half of all diseased teeth are concentrated in just 7% of five-year-olds serves to highlight the health inequalities that pervade our society. It is crucial that from the earliest stage of their training, the next generation of dental professionals have an appreciation that the lives of others are frequently very different from their own.

Dental students rightly spend the majority of their time learning the theoretical, practical and clinical skills necessary to practise their chosen profession. Often it is only relatively late in their course that their attention turns to the environment in which they will have to deliver dental care and earn their living. It is important to have an appreciation of the issues involved in the organisation, commissioning and delivery of oral healthcare at dental practice, regional, national and international levels. The principles of evidence-based practice are of ever-increasing significance in achieving this. In its guidance Preparing for Practice, the General Dental Council has placed great emphasis on learning outcomes that fall within the remit of dental public health. All of these factors emphasise the need for an understanding of the discipline.

The intention of this book is that 'at a glance' dental professionals will be able to come to a basic understanding of the principles and practice that relate to the science and the art of improving oral health at both an individual and a population level. Of course, the factors influencing public health practice evolve at a pace – a change of government, new guidance and new policies affect dental public health at a greater rate than other dental specialties. For this reason, the intention of this book is to raise awareness and provide pointers and flags that can be followed up via more exhaustive information sources.

While the basic principles of the discipline are universal, a complicating factor in writing a book on dental public health in the United Kingdom is the four different – sometimes very different – models of care that have evolved in the constituent countries following devolution in 1999. Where possible, attempts have been made to illustrate differences across the United Kingdom, but at times this is limited by the constraints of space.

The primary audience for this book is undergraduate dental, dental therapy and dental hygiene students, together with those in Dental Foundation and Core training and those preparing for MDFS or MJDF examinations. The book should also prove a useful resource for those preparing for the Diploma in Dental Public Health examination or the Overseas Registration examination. While at an entry level, the book may also act as an aide-memoire for those undertaking specialty training, and may indeed be of use to any member of the dental team who has an interest in the vast range of topics now embraced within dental public health.

The concepts arising in dental public health can be challenging from an academic perspective. Twenty years teaching the subject have taught me that it is one that students tend to love or hate. It is my hope that this book might go some way to encouraging more of the former and less of the latter.

Ivor G. Chestnutt
Cardiff
April 2015

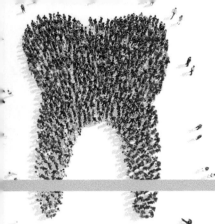

Preface to the second edition

Many years ago, when I was a trainee in dental public a senior manager wrote on the blackboard, 'the only thing constant in public health is change'. How true that has proven in the eight years since I wrote the first edition of this book.

As a basic text, the fundamentals of epidemiology, study design, evidence-based practice, measuring and recording oral health and dental disease remain the same. However, who would have thought that a situation would arise in which for months, routine dental care was suspended? The COVID-19 pandemic brought the discipline of public health to the fore with senior public health practitioners appearing alongside the most senior politicians on television, night after night. In updating this book, a new chapter on pandemics and their relevance to dental practice has been added. The other ever-increasing and significant threat to human health is that posed by global climate change. A new chapter discusses the environmental agenda and its implications for dental practice.

In the time since the first edition there have also been advances in how we plan and think about facilitating behaviour change and an additional chapter on that topic has also been included. In the field of health improvement we have seen the introduction of fiscal measures to control the intake of drinks high in free sugars as well as minimum pricing of alcohol in some parts of the United Kingdom, both policies that are likely to benefit oral health.

Access to NHS dentistry has been a particular issue, because of not only the pandemic but also the mechanisms used to contract for the provision of dental services. These issues are discussed as are the various attempts to reform the contract for delivery of NHS dental care.

Internationally, the World Health Organization has produced a global oral health strategy, incorporating the concept of universal health coverage and this is discussed in detail.

Of course, underlying all of the above are the inequalities that persist in the experience of oral disease across society, a paradigm not helped by the 'cost of living' crisis that has impacted so many.

As I said in the introduction to the first edition of this textbook, it is crucial that the dental professionals of tomorrow have a view of how lifestyle, life circumstances and social factors will impact on the communities in which they will eventually practice. I hope that this second edition continues to deliver the basics of Dental Public Health and enthuses and inspires further cohorts of those pursuing a career in dentistry.

Ivor G. Chestnutt
Cardiff
October 2023

Introduction

Part 1

Chapters

1   What is dental public health?

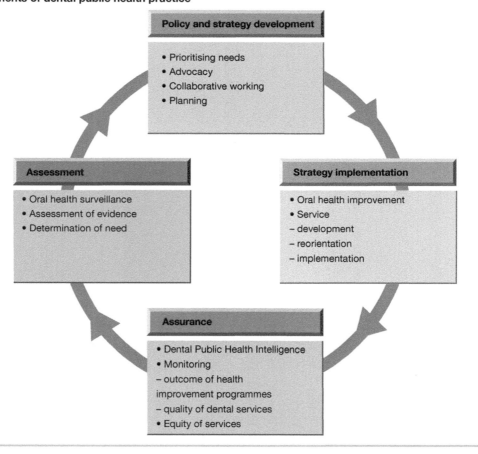

Figure 1.1   The essential elements of dental public health. Source: *Adapted from a diagram produced by the British Association for the Study of Community Dentistry.*

Health improvement	Healthcare public health	Health protection	Health intelligence	Workforce development	Academic public health
Improving health across populations and systems	Relates to the organisation of dental services to ensure effective and efficient delivery of dental care	Providing advice on the control of infection and management of health and safety in oral healthcare	Analysis of epidemiological, clinical and dental service information	Strategic planning and development of dental and dental public health workforce	Research and education

Figure 1.2   Components of dental public health practice

Policy and strategy development
- Prioritising needs
- Advocacy
- Collaborative working
- Planning

Assessment
- Oral health surveillance
- Assessment of evidence
- Determination of need

Strategy implementation
- Oral health improvement
- Service
- development
- reorientation
- implementation

Assurance
- Dental Public Health Intelligence
- Monitoring
- outcome of health improvement programmes
- quality of dental services
- Equity of services

In contrast to clinical dental practice, where the focus is on looking after individual patients, in dental public health practice, the focus is on populations or defined groups within a population. As outlined in Table 1.1, the definition refers to **science**. Dental public health requires a sound knowledge of the factors influencing the aetiology, detection, measurement, description and prevention of oral disease, as well as the promotion of oral health. It also refers to **art**. This involves advocacy, policy development and the politics of how

dental care is prioritised, organised, monitored and paid for in societies.

The essential elements of dental public health are shown in Figure 1.1.

The key components of dental public health practice and how these relate to one another are shown in Figure 1.2. The core values of public health practice are as in Table 1.2.

A comparison between clinical dental practice and dental public health practice is shown in Table 1.3.

Table 1.1 Definition of dental public health

Dental public health is the science and the art of preventing oral disease, promoting oral health and improving the quality of life through the organised efforts of society.

Table 1.2 Core values of public health practice, as defined by the Faculty of Public Health in the UK

- Equitable
- Empowering
- Effective
- Evidence-based
- Fair
- Inclusive

Table 1.3 A comparison between clinical dental practice and dental public health

Individual clinical practice	Public health practice
Individual patients	Populations and defined groups within populations
Examination	Epidemiology, surveys
Diagnosis	Assessment of need
Treatment planning	Prioritisation and programme planning
Informed consent for treatment	Ethics and planning approval
An appropriate mix of care, cure and prevention	Programme implementation
Payment for services	Programme budgeting/finance
Evaluation	Appraisal and review

Table 1.4 The public health approach as applied to dentistry

Dental public health:
- Is concerned with the oral health of populations
  - in a city or defined geographical area
  - in a particular group of the population defined by a common demographic, e.g. children, older people
  - in a group of people with social circumstances in common, e.g. homeless people, people with drug and substance abuse problems.
- Recognises that responsibility for health and prevention of oral disease is shared between individuals and healthcare professionals and that people should be empowered to look after their own health.
- Is conscious that as health is markedly linked to people's lifestyles and life circumstances, it needs to take account of how the risk of poor oral health is not equal across populations, e.g. levels of dental caries in children are closely correlated with social and economic deprivation.
- It implies that to improve health, it is necessary to work on policy development at a high level and across disciplines. As an example, legislation making the wearing of seat belts compulsory is important in preventing facial injuries in road traffic accidents; taxing tobacco sales is important in moderating smoking. In health improvement programmes in schools, dental public health practitioners need to work outside of health and collaborate with school teachers and education authorities.

The public health approach

The Faculty of Public Health, the professional body that is responsible for setting standards in public health practice in the UK, describes the public health approach as follows:
- population-based
- emphasising collective responsibility for health, its protection and disease prevention
- recognising the key role of the state, linked to a concern for the underlying socio-economic and wider determinants of health, as well as disease
- emphasising partnerships with all those who contribute to the health of the population.

How this applies to dental public health is shown in Table 1.4.

Key disciplines in dental public health

In order to practise dental public health, knowledge of the following disciplines is important.

Oral epidemiology

Oral epidemiology is the study of oral health and oral disease and their determinants in populations.

Demography

This refers to measurements and statistics that describe populations. It involves recording factors such as the age structure, ethnic composition and educational attainment of the population.

Medical statistics

Understanding numbers and the inferences that can be drawn from them is a key skill in reviewing disease trends and service provision, as is the ability to appraise and conduct dental research.

Health promotion and health improvement

Health promotion is the process of enabling people to increase control over their health and its determinants, thereby improving their health. Health improvement recognises that the determinants of health can be outside an individual's control and is designed to address so-called wider determinants of health such as education, housing and employment. It is also designed to address the gaps in health between areas of high and low social and economic provision – gaps known as 'health inequalities'.

Sociology

Sociology is the study of the development, structure and functioning of human societies. Understanding these factors is important in improving health and organising healthcare services.

Psychology

Psychology is the branch of science that deals with the human mind and its functions. In a public health context, understanding psychology is important in relation to behaviour change.

Health economics

Health economics concerns the need for, demand for and supply of health and healthcare. In dental public health, it relates to how resources are distributed and the effectiveness and efficiency of services. Understanding how care is commissioned and paid for is an important element of how dentistry is organised and delivered, and dental public health practitioners need a clear understanding of these issues.

Health services management and planning

Dental services compete with other forms of healthcare, whether paid for by the state or individuals. They, therefore need to be organised, managed and planned. The allocation of resources within a publicly funded dental service should be proportional to the need and likelihood of benefit. Dental public health practitioners will be called on to give advice to health service managers and finance officers on the appropriate allocation of resources and to offer guidance on how dental services are planned and delivered.

Evidence-based practice

Evidence-based practice is designed to ensure that, wherever possible, the dental care that is delivered has been shown to be the most efficient and effective. It is the role of dental public health practitioners to facilitate such practice. Those responsible for dental public health need to understand the theory of evidence-based dentistry to support the improvement of oral health and the delivery of effective care.

2 Health, oral health and their determinants

Figure 2.1 The determinants of health. Source: *Adapted from Dahlgren and Whitehead (1991). Reproduced with permission from the Institute for Futures Studies.*

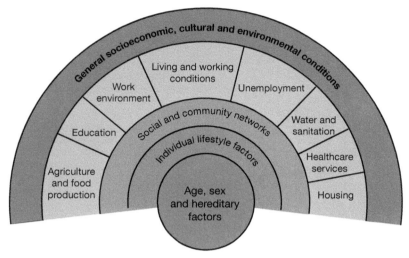

Figure 2.2 Life circumstances and lifestyle as determinants of health

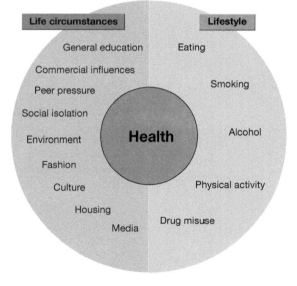

Figure 2.3 Lifecourse analysis as a means of investigating the determinants of health

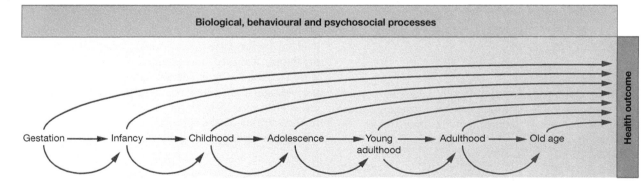

Health

The most widely accepted definition of health is that offered by the World Health Organization in 1948, which states:

Health is a complete state of physical, mental and social wellbeing and not merely the absence of disease or infirmity.

The key point in this definition is that health is more than simply not being ill. It encompasses all aspects of an individual's being. Today, health is also recognised as not solely a desired state to acquire, but a means to enable individuals to live their lives to the full and 'be all they can be'.

Oral health

Mirroring the definition of general health, oral health can be defined as follows:

Oral health is a standard of health of the oral and related tissues without active disease. That state should enable the individual to eat, speak and socialise without discomfort or embarrassment and contribute to general wellbeing.

This means that while a patient may have no active dental decay or periodontal disease, if they are embarrassed by the appearance of their teeth when they smile, they cannot be said to have true oral health. This definition also recognises that good oral health is integral to overall health. Older people who cannot eat properly because they lack sufficient teeth or have inadequate dentures may become nutritionally compromised.

The impact of oral disease on individuals can be measured using social-dental indicators as presented in Chapter 4.

Determinants of health and oral health

Determinant simply means 'factor influencing'. Many things can influence health. The diagram in Figure 2.1 was drawn by Dahlgren and Whitehead in 1991. It illustrates the concept of health being influenced by factors that operate at different levels.

Innate determinants of health

First, health is determined by factors innate to the individual. So age, gender and genetic makeup will all influence health. These determinants are not easily amenable to change. For example, a degree of attachment loss and periodontal recession is almost inevitable as a patient ages. However, this will probably reflect a mixture of ageing and exposure to the next level of determinants, such as lifestyle.

Lifestyle as a determinant of health

Health and oral health can be markedly influenced by lifestyle. Diet, smoking, consumption of alcohol and lack of exercise all have the potential to impact health. Dental caries is caused by exposure to excess fermentable carbohydrates (sugars), and tobacco smoking is a significant risk factor in the aetiology of periodontal disease and oral cancer (Figure 2.2).

Life circumstances as determinants of health

While lifestyle can be thought of as things people do to themselves (behaviours), life circumstances are things that happen to people and are, to a large degree, outside their direct control. For example, peer pressure may lead a teenager to feel compelled to have an intra-oral piercing, or advertising may persuade people to consume foods high in sugar (Figure 2.2).

Social and community networks as determinants of health

Interaction with others and the support that they provide are recognised as important determinants of health. Peer support and social interaction are necessary components of health for most people.

General socio-economic, cultural and environmental conditions as determinants of health

At the highest level, social and economic factors have a major influence on health. Policies decided at national and international levels have impacts on health. The ability of a community or country to provide basic education for its population, for example, will have an impact on health literacy. The proportion of a country's gross domestic product (GDP, i.e. the country's wealth) that is devoted to health services can influence the ease of access to medical and dental care. There are large variations in the proportion of national wealth that is spent on health in different countries. In 2019, the United States spent 16.8% of GDP on healthcare, while the United Kingdom devoted 10.2% and France spent 11.1%. In developing countries, the proportion of national wealth spent on health services is typically low, of the order of 3–5%, while at the same time, vast sums are often spent on military and defence services.

The impact of the environment on health is of major concern. Worldwide issues such as global warming have significant implications for health. However, even at present, environmental issues can influence health and oral health. Over-exposure to sunshine and lack of use of protective sunscreens can cause skin cancers in the head and neck region. Conversely, underexposure to sunshine can result in a lack of vitamin D and diseases such as rickets.

Lifecourse analysis

This approach to understanding the determinants of health looks at how events in early life or across generations can affect susceptibility to disease in adulthood. Lifecourse studies investigate biological, psychological and behavioural factors and how these operate during gestation, childhood, adolescence and young adulthood to influence disease in later life (Figure 2.3). These types of studies involve following up a cohort of people over time. An example is the Dunedin Multidisciplinary Health and Development study. In this study, a pool of children born in the Otago Region in New Zealand in 1972 and 1973 was recruited and examined at ages 3, 5, 7, 9, 11, 13, 15, 18, 21, 26, 32, 38 and, most recently, at age 45 (2017–2019). Oral health has been investigated as part of this study.

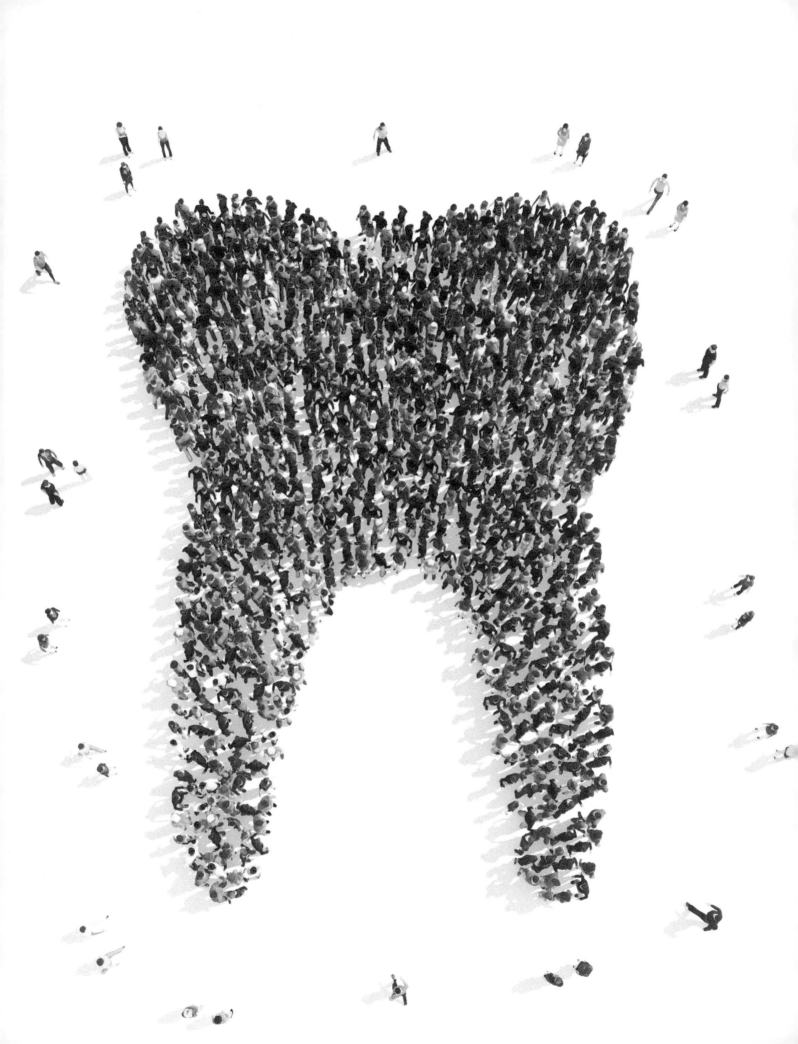

Epidemiology

Part 2

Chapters

3 Basic epidemiology

Figure 3.1   What is epidemiology?

Epidemiology is the study of the distribution and determinants of diseases and injuries in populations

– distribution = location
– determinant = cause or risk factor

Figure 3.2   The principle components of an epidemiological study

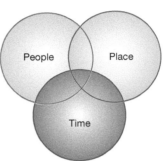

Figure 3.3   Age and sex of the population, 2011–2021, England and Wales. Source: *Reproduced with permission from the Office for National Statistics.*

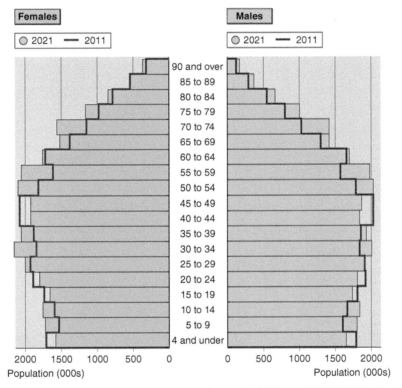

Epidemiology

Epidemiology, from 'epi' =about and 'demos' =people, is the branch of science that deals with the study of the distribution of health and illness and their determinants (or influencing factors) in populations or groups of people at a particular time or over a period of time (Figure 3.1).

Thus, three key elements can be identified in an epidemiological study: people, place and time (Figure 3.2).

Describing disease in populations

Count data

The simplest measure in an epidemiological study is a count of the number of people in an area affected by a particular condition at one point in time. For example, it is possible to state that there were x people affected by oral cancer in a given country on a given day (assuming we could accurately identify and count this). This information can be used to plan services. However, counting data on their own is of limited value. This is because they do not contain denominator data. That means it is unknown how many people have the condition out of those who could be affected. So, in the oral cancer example, simply reporting the number of people with oral cancer gives no idea of whether a large or small proportion of the population is affected. It would not be possible to identify changes over time (as the number of people at risk may change) or to make comparisons between different areas or countries. For this reason, data in epidemiology are almost always reported as rates or proportions.

Prevalence

One of the most common ways of describing the amount of disease in a population is by reporting the prevalence.

*Prevalence is the proportion of people with a disease at any given point (**point prevalence**) or period (**period prevalence**) in time.*

Incidence

While prevalence describes the amount of disease present at a given point or period, incidence describes the amount of new disease that occurs over a given period of time.

Incidence is the number of new cases of a disease in a defined population over a defined period of time. Incidence measures events – a change from a healthy to a diseased state.

It is important to remember these terms and use them correctly. In common usage, for example, in the press and media, the terms prevalence and incidence are frequently employed incorrectly and interchangeably without regard to their correct meaning.

Standardised data

Standardisation is a technique that is used to account for the effect of confounding factors in populations.

Oral cancer is more common in older people and men. Suppose we are interested in deaths due to oral cancer, age and gender act as confounding factors. As a result, when comparing deaths from oral cancer between two cities, it is important to take into account the age and gender structure of those communities. For example, a city with a large student population would have a different age and gender structure than a seaside town where many older people have retired.

Standardised mortality ratio (SMR)

To overcome this problem and allow comparison of deaths due to oral cancer, taking into account confounding factors, a standardised mortality ratio (SMR) is calculated:

$$\text{Standardised mortality ratio}\,(\text{SMR}) = (\text{Observed deaths} / \text{Expected deaths})$$

To do this, the deaths in a particular area are compared with a wider population. In the aforementioned case, we could calculate the deaths in different age bands for males and females in the whole country. This constitutes the expected deaths. We could also calculate the deaths in these same age bands and by gender in our university city or seaside town. This is the observed death rate. The actual or observed number of deaths can then be compared with the expected number. The ratio of observed to expected deaths gives the mortality ratio and is usually expressed as a percentage. The mortality ratio in the whole county is 100 (because the number of expected and observed deaths is, by definition, the same). If the resulting value is greater than 100, that would indicate that oral cancer-related mortality was unfavourable, even having accounted for the age and gender structure of the population. A value of less than 100 indicates a more favourable mortality.

Demography

Demography is the scientific discipline that studies populations and how they are affected by factors such as births, deaths, gender, age structure and migration. Population structure can be represented by a population pyramid, such as that shown in Figure 3.3. The population is plotted in five-year age bands, with numbers of females on the left and numbers of males on the right. The shape can be used to deduce a population's relative number of old and young people. The UK population structure is typical of a Western developed country, where the top of the pyramid is relatively broad, indicating a low young: old person ratio. A population pyramid for a developing country would have a much broader base and more steeply sloping sides, indicating a high young: old person ratio.

Increased longevity and a greater number of older people in the UK population have seen the ratio of young to old people decrease in recent years. The age structure can also be affected by migration. Migrants tend to be young and have more children. Health service planners need to make provision for such population changes.

4 Principles of measuring and recording oral disease and oral health

Table 4.1 Common dental indices and the conditions they measure

Index	Condition measured
DMFT/dmft (decayed, missing and filled)	Dental caries
ICDAS – International Caries Detection and Assessment System	Dental caries
Significant caries index (based on DMFT/dmft)	Dental caries
Root caries index	Root caries
Community Periodontal Index of Treatment Need (CPITN) – Basic Periodontal Examination (BPE)	Periodontal disease
Plaque index	Dental plaque
Modified gingival index	Gingivitis
IOTN (Index of Orthodontic Treatment Need)	Orthodontic treatment need
PAR (Peer Assessment Rating)	Orthodontic treatment outcome
Erosion index	Erosion/non-carious tooth surface loss
Dean's index	Fluorosis
Modified DDE	Developmental defects of enamel

Table 4.2 Interpretation of the strength of agreement determined by kappa (κ) statistic

Value of κ	Strength of agreement
1.00–0.81	Very good
0.80–0.61	Good
0.60–0.41	Moderate
0.40–0.21	Fair
<0.20	Poor

Table 4.3 Reasons for measuring and recording oral disease

At an INDIVIDUAL level	At a POPULATION level
Clinical management	
To aid diagnosis	To record the prevalence of disease in a population
To aid treatment	To aid understanding of the aetiology of diseases
To measure individual treatment need	To provide an indication of population treatment need
To measure individual treatment outcome	To evaluate the effectiveness of public health programmes
Research (e.g. in clinical trials)	
To test the effect of new treatments or products	

Table 4.4 Oral Health Impact Profile 14 (OHIP 14)

Dimension	Question – How often in the last 12 months
Functional limitation	Have you had trouble *pronouncing any words* because of problems with your mouth teeth or dentures?
	Have you felt that your *sense of taste* has worsened because of problems with your mouth teeth or dentures?
Physical pain	Have you had *painful aching* in your mouth?
	Have you found it *uncomfortable to eat any foods* because of problems with your teeth, mouth or dentures?
Psychological discomfort	Have you been *self-conscious* because of your teeth, mouth or dentures?
	Have you *felt tense* because of problems with your mouth teeth or dentures?
Physical disability	Has your *diet been unsatisfactory* because of problems with your mouth teeth or dentures?
	Have you had to *interrupt meals* because of problems with your mouth teeth or dentures?
Psychological disability	Have you found it *difficult to relax* because of problems with your mouth teeth or dentures?
	Have you been a bit *embarrassed* because of problems with your mouth teeth or dentures?
Social disability	Have you been a bit *irritable with other people* because of problems with your mouth teeth or dentures?
	Have you had *difficulty doing your usual jobs* because of problems with your mouth teeth or dentures?
Handicap	Have you felt that life in general was *less satisfying* because of problems with your mouth teeth or dentures?
	Have you been *totally unable to function* because of problems with your mouth teeth or dentures?

Responses on a 5-point scale coded 0 = never, 1 = hardly ever, 2 = occasionally, 3 = fairly often, 4 = very often.

Source: *Slade (1997)/John Wiley & Sons.*

Dental Public Health at a Glance, Second Edition. Ivor G. Chestnutt.
© 2024 John Wiley & Sons Ltd. Published 2024 by John Wiley & Sons Ltd.

What is a dental index?

To record the presence, extent and severity of dental disease in a consistent manner, a suitable method is required. Such recording systems are termed dental indices (singular: dental index). Over the years, numerous dental indices have been developed, and standardised ways of recording most dental conditions and pathologies exist. Examples of commonly used dental indices are shown in Table 4.1.

The properties of an ideal dental index

An ideal dental index should have the following features:

• **Simple:** The index should be simple to understand and easy to learn. This is important if large numbers of clinicians are to be taught how to use the index consistently. It should also be simple to administer. An index that takes a long time to record reduces the efficiency of collecting data in epidemiological surveys, where clinicians need to record a large amount of data in a short period of time.

• **Objective:** There should be as little scope as possible for subjective interpretation on the part of the examining clinician. This limits the chances of different clinicians recording different levels of disease when examining identical clinical conditions.

• **Clear-cut categories:** The division between categories or codes used within an index should be clear. It is also helpful if these categories relate to distinct stages of the clinical condition being measured. If these distinct stages are associated to different treatment needs, then it is possible to construct an index that not only measures the presence of a disease, but can also give an indication of treatment needs Common examples include the community periodontal index of treatment need (CPITN) and the index of orthodontic treatment need (IOTN).

• **Valid:** The index must measure what it is intended to measure. For example, an index designed to measure early dental decay (white spots) must not be confused by developmental hypoplasia (which can also appear as a white/demineralised spot).

• **Reliable:** Each time the index is used, it should record the same outcome (provided the disease remains the same). This relates to the properties of the index.

• **Reproducible:** Each time the index is used, it should record the same outcome, either when two different examiners use the index to measure the same condition (inter-examiner reproducibility) or when the same examiner measures the condition on two different occasions (intra-examiner reproducibility). This is provided, of course, that the condition being measured has not changed between examinations. The degree of agreement between or within examiners is measured statistically using the Kappa statistic (κ). This is a more robust measure than simply calculating the percentage agreement between examiners, as κ takes into account agreement that has occurred by chance. The Kappa statistic is reported as a value between 0 and 1 and is interpreted as shown in Table 4.2.

• **Quantifiable:** It is an advantage if the output of a dental index is amenable to statistical analysis.

• **Sensitive:** An ideal index should be able to detect and record small changes in levels of disease.

• **Reversible:** A good index should respond to improvements in the measured dental condition.

• **Future risk:** It is an advantage if a dental index can give an indication of the future risk of disease.

Few dental indices meet all of these ideal characteristics.

Why is it necessary to measure and record dental disease?

Measuring dental diseases can be viewed from two perspectives: in the context of measuring disease either in an individual in a clinical context or in an individual as part of a population group. The reasons for measuring in these contexts are described in Table 4.3.

Many dental indices were initially developed for use in research studies (e.g. plaque and gingivitis indices) and then subsequently used in clinical treatment settings. Other indices employed in the diagnosis and clinical management of patients were derived from indices initially developed for use in epidemiological surveys. For instance, the Basic Periodontal Examination (BPE) evolved from the Community Periodontal Index of Treatment Need CPITN.

Socio-dental indicators of oral health

The dental indicators described in Table 4.1 measure dental diseases from a normative perspective. This means that the disease is mainly judged from a clinician's perspective. Therefore, these indices do not capture the full impact of the disease on the patient in terms of how they function or the impact of the disease on their general health or on their lifestyle and daily living. A range of indices called socio-dental indicators have been developed to capture the impact of dental and oral disease beyond the mainly physical signs and symptoms on which traditional indices rely.

A commonly used socio-dental indicator is the Oral Health Impact Profile (OHIP). This comprised 49 questions when originally devised, but a more user-friendly version with just 14 questions has been developed (OHIP-14; see Table 4.4). This asks two questions on each of the seven dimensions of impact. Patients are asked using a five-point scale how commonly they have experienced these impacts in the past 12 months, and a score is derived. This can be used to compare the impact with population norms or to investigate the effect of providing different forms of treatment.

5 Epidemiology of dental caries

Figure 5.1 The DMF/dmf index for recording dental caries

D/d = decay M/m = missing F/f = filled

DMF – refers to the *permanent* dentition

dmf – refers to the *primary* dentition

DMFT – refers to teeth and indicates the number of permanent teeth, filled, missing or decayed. Can score 0–32 (0–28 if exclude 3rd molars).

dmft indicates the number of primary teeth, filled, missing or decayed. Can score 0–20

DMFS – refers to the number of surfaces of permanent teeth filled, missing or decayed. If missing due to caries: Incisors and canines count as 4 surfaces, premolars and molars as 5

DMFS can score 0–148 (0–128 if exclude 3rd molars)

dmfs can score 0–88

Components of DMF can be used to determine:

$$\frac{D}{DMF} = \text{index of treatment need}$$

$$\frac{F}{DMF} = \text{Index of treatment provision (or Care Index)}$$

$$\frac{M}{DMF} = \text{index of treatment failure}$$

Figure 5.2 Extent of dental decay as defined in conventional dental epidemiology surveys

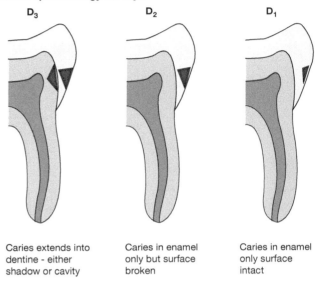

D_3	D_2	D_1
Caries extends into dentine - either shadow or cavity	Caries in enamel only but surface broken	Caries in enamel only surface intact

Figure 5.3 Calculation of the significant caries index

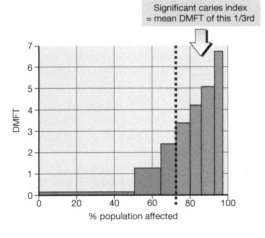

Significant caries index = mean DMFT of this 1/3rd

Figure 5.4 Obvious dental decay in 15-year-olds in the UK 1973–2013

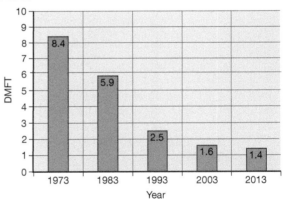

Figure 5.5 Schematic representation of changes in the distribution of dental caries in children in the United Kingdom between 1970 and 2023

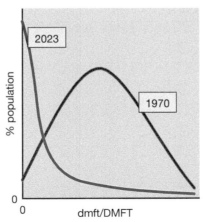

Dental Public Health at a Glance, Second Edition. Ivor G. Chestnutt.
© 2024 John Wiley & Sons Ltd. Published 2024 by John Wiley & Sons Ltd.

Recording dental caries in oral health surveys

The DMF/dmf Index

Dental caries is recorded using the DMF/dmf Index. This records the number of teeth that are decayed, missing or filled as a result of dental caries (DMFT/dmft) or the number of tooth surfaces (DMFS/dmfs) similarly affected. Conventions for the use of the index are shown in Figure 5.1.

Decay can be scored at the D1, D2 and D3 levels (Figure 5.2). Traditionally, dental surveys and clinical trials worldwide have been conducted using the DMF Index, with caries scored at the D3 level or into dentine. Increasingly studies also report caries prevalence at the D1 and D2 levels (enamel caries). It is important to establish what threshold is being used when discussing caries prevalence – at the dentinal or into enamel level.

The components of the index can be used to calculate treatment needs, provision and failure.

ICDAS International Caries Detection and Assessment System

This index uses two scores per tooth surface. The first code relates to the restorative status of the tooth, and the second to the caries status. The ICDAS index was developed primarily to enable the degree of caries' progress into dental enamel to be recorded in greater detail than is possible with the traditional DMF Index. Full details of the index can be found on the ICDAS website (www.icdas.org).

Significant Caries Index

This index was developed to take account of the skewed distribution of dental caries in populations. The large proportion of caries-free individuals can mask the true extent of caries in affected individuals by reducing the population mean (Figure 5.3). To calculate the Significant Caries Index, individuals are sorted according to their DMFT values. The third of the population with the highest caries score is selected, and the mean DMFT for this subgroup is calculated.

Epidemiological surveys for dental caries

There is a long history of oral health surveys in the United Kingdom.

Decennial surveys

Between 1968 and 2013, a series of surveys of the oral health of adults and children has been conducted every 10 years. Until the most recent surveys, these covered all of the United Kingdom. However, following the devolution of responsibility for health to Northern Ireland, Scotland and Wales administrations there have instituted their own dental epidemiology/inspection programmes as a means of surveying oral health in children. As a result, the UK national surveys have ceased.

'BASCD surveys'

In addition to the decennial surveys, local health bodies conducted a long-standing series of surveys of children's oral health across the United Kingdom in collaboration with the British Association for the Study of Community Dentistry (BASCD). These are evolving into distinct programmes within the four countries in the United Kingdom.

The decennial and BASCD surveys have provided key information for oral health needs assessment and dental service planning.

Caries prevalence in the United Kingdom

Children

Figure 5.4 shows changes in the prevalence of dental caries in 15-year-olds. This illustrates the remarkable improvement that oral health has seen in the United Kingdom in the past half-century. It is difficult for the current generation of dental students to appreciate a time when half of all 15-year-olds had eight or more decayed permanent teeth. The changes observed can largely be attributed to the introduction of fluoride-containing toothpaste, which became widely available from the early 1970s onwards.

Adults

The number of sound untreated teeth by age in England is shown in Table 5.1. From this, it is apparent that the mean number of teeth unaffected by dental caries increased across all age groups between 1978 and 2009. There have been no UK adult dental health surveys since 2009. Changes in the pattern of tooth loss in adults are shown in Figure 9.1.

Changes in the distribution of dental caries in the population

An important change in how dental caries is distributed across the population occurred as oral health improved. In the early 1970s, dental caries in children was normally distributed; that is, while a small number of the population were caries-free, the majority of the population experienced decay to a greater or lesser degree. As oral health improved, the caries-free proportion of the population increased, but the disease burden fell on a smaller proportion of the population. The distribution of the disease became skewed (Figure 5.5). Those affected by caries increasingly were from more deprived social and economic circumstances (Chapter 19). This gives rise to the concept of a 'high-risk' group in the population.

Table 5.1 Mean number of sound and untreated teeth by age in England, 1978–2009

Age (years)	1978	1988	1998	2009
16–24	17.5	21.7	23.7	26.1
25–34	14.1	16.4	19.5	24.0
35–44	12.4	13.3	15.9	20.4
45–54	10.6	11.7	11.9	15.2
55–64	9.2	9.5	9.7	12.0
65+			8.6	9.6
All	13.2	15.0	15.6	18.0

N.B. The criteria changed after 1998. No comparable data are available beyond 2009 due to changes in survey methodology.
Source: *Data from Health and Social Care Information Centre (2011).*

6 Epidemiology of periodontal disease

Figure 6.1 **Common plaque and gingival indices.** Source: *Data from Greene and Vermillion (1960); from Silness and Löe (1964); and Löe (1967).*

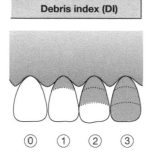

| Debris index (DI) | Silness and Löe (1964) | Löe (1967) |

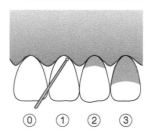

**Debris index
(Greene and Vermillion 1960)**

0 = No plaque

1 = Plaque covering 1/3 tooth

2 = Plaque covering 2/3 tooth

3 = Plaque totally covering tooth

**Plaque index
(Silness and Löe 1964)**

0 = No plaque detected

1 = Looks clean but material can be
removed from gingival third with probe

2 = Visible plaque

3 = Tooth covered with abundant plaque

**Modified gingival index
(Löe 1967)**

0 = Healthy gingivae

1 = Gingivae look inflamed,
but don't bleed when probed

2 = Gingivae look inflamed
and bleed when probed

3 = Ulceration and spontaneous bleeding

Figure 6.2 **Periodontal health by age group, UK 2009.** Source: *Data from Health and Social Care Information Centre (2011).*

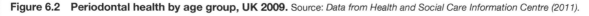
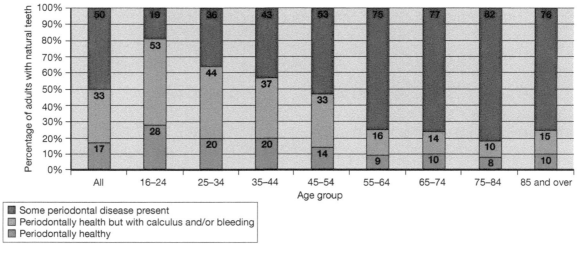

- ■ Some periodontal disease present
- ■ Periodontally health but with calculus and/or bleeding
- ■ Periodontally healthy

Periodontal disease includes all pathological conditions of the periodontium, but commonly refers to inflammatory conditions induced by dental plaque – namely, gingivitis and periodontitis. Gingivitis is an inflammatory response of the gingivae without the destruction of the tooth-supporting apparatus. Periodontitis results in destruction of the fibres and bone that support the tooth and initially presents as the development of a periodontal pocket. Diseases affecting the periodontal tissues are classified as shown in Table 6.1.

Periodontal indices

In measuring the prevalence of periodontal disease, the primary clinical features that are recorded are the presence and amount of dental plaque and calculus, inflammation of the gingivae, presence and depth of periodontal pockets, attachment loss (pocket depth plus recession) and mobility of teeth. Numerous periodontal indices have been developed to measure these features (Figure 6.1). The community periodontal index of treatment need (CPITN) was developed by the World Health Organization. The mouth is divided into sextants (two posterior and one anterior per arch), and the worst score per sextant is recorded (Table 6.2). This was subsequently adapted to form the basic periodontal examination for use in clinical settings.

Susceptibility to periodontitis

The prevalence of periodontal pocketing increases with age, but severe periodontitis affects only 10–15% of the population. The prevalence of severe periodontitis worldwide is reported in Figure 10.2.

Dental Public Health at a Glance, Second Edition. Ivor G. Chestnutt.
© 2024 John Wiley & Sons Ltd. Published 2024 by John Wiley & Sons Ltd.

Table 6.1 Classification scheme for periodontal and peri-implant diseases and conditions (2017)

1. Health
   - Intact periodontium
   - Reduced periodontium
2. Plaque-induced gingivitis: (localised/generalised gingivitis)
   - Intact periodontium
   - Reduced periodontium
3. Non plaque-induced gingival disease and conditions
4. Periodontitis
   - Localised (<30% teeth)
   - Generalised (>30% teeth)
   - Molar-incisor pattern
5. Necrotising periodontal diseases
6. Periodontitis as a manifestation of systemic diseases
7. Systemic disease or conditions affecting the periodontal tissues
8. Periodontal abscesses
9. Periodontal-endodontic lesions
10. Mucogingival deformities and conditions

Table 6.2 Community periodontal index treatment need (CPITN) scores

CPITN score	Clinical parameters
Code 0	Healthy, no pockets >3.5 mm, no bleeding on probing, no calculus, no defective restoration margins
Code 1	No pockets >3.5 mm, bleeding on probing but no calculus, no defective restoration margins
Code 2	No pockets >3.5 mm, bleeding on probing and either calculus or defective restoration margins
Code 3	Pockets >3.5 mm <5.5 mm
Code 4	Pockets >5.5 mm

Periodontal health in the United Kingdom

In a 2018 survey of adults attending general dental practices in England, just over half of the participants had gingival bleeding on gentle probing (52.9%). More men (56.5%) than women (50.4%) had gingival bleeding. There was no clear pattern in gingival bleeding by age and little variation by ethnic group. Participants living in the most deprived areas of the country were more likely (60.4%) to have gingival bleeding than participants living in the least deprived areas (46.9%). Participants who had last attended the dentist two or more years ago were more likely (60.9%) to have gingival bleeding than participants who had last attended less than two years ago (52.1%).

The 2018 survey did not probe to determine periodontal pockets. The most recent data on the prevalence of periodontitis in the United Kingdom comes from the last Adult Dental Health Survey in 2009. The authors of that survey reported periodontal status as:
- **Periodontally healthy** – Defined as no bleeding, no calculus, no pocketing or loss of attachment greater than 4 mm.
- Periodontally healthy but with calculus or bleeding, no pockets or loss of attachment greater than 4 mm.
- Some periodontal disease is present, with pocketing of 4 mm or more.

Overall, just 17% of adults were deemed to be totally periodontally healthy; that is, no pockets >4 mm and no bleeding or calculus. The prevalence of periodontal disease increased with age, such that from age 55 and over, at least 75% of the population had a periodontal pocket or attachment loss of at least 4 mm at one or more sites (Figure 6.2).

While the prevalence of periodontal pockets increases with age, only a small proportion of the population experiences periodontal disease at a level that will cause them to lose a large number of teeth.

Oral cleanliness and oral hygiene practices

In the 2009 UK Adult Dental Health Survey, two-thirds (66%) of adults had dental plaque present on at least one tooth, and there were on average, six teeth on which plaque deposits could be detected. A similar proportion (68%) had calculus present in at least one sextant of their mouths.

In this survey, 75% of adults claimed to brush their teeth twice per day. Women were more likely to do so than men (82% versus 67%). A further 23% of the population claimed to brush their teeth once a day. Only 2% reported brushing less than once per day, and 1% suggested that they never brushed their teeth.

An association was observed between the frequency of tooth brushing and socioeconomic status. While 79% of adults from managerial and professional backgrounds said they brushed their teeth twice a day, in routine and manual occupation households, the corresponding figure was 68%.

The use of other products to clean teeth was reported by 58% of dentate adults, with mouthwash (31%), electric toothbrushes (26%) and dental floss (21%) being the most frequently cited.

Predisposing and modifying (risk) factors for periodontal disease

Individuals are not equally at risk of developing periodontal disease. Local and systemic risk factors are shown in Table 6.3.

Periodontal disease and systemic disease

A great deal of research effort has been expended on determining the possible effect of periodontal disease on general health. Studies suggest that periodontal health impacts systemic health and vice versa. Links with a long list of diseases and conditions, including cardiovascular disease, chronic kidney disease, diabetes, pulmonary disease, prostate cancer, colon cancer, pancreatic cancer, preterm pregnancy, erectile dysfunction, Alzheimer's disease and rheumatoid arthritis have all been reported. The most important open question related to these associations is causality. The pathophysiological mechanism, cause-effect, or dose-response relationships are still unclear. Confounding (i.e. the role of intermediate or underlying factors) remains the most challenging issue in interpreting the associations found. The results of studies are often contradictory and lack homogeneity. The true nature of the impact of periodontal disease on general health awaits determination.

Table 6.3 Predisposing and modifying factors in susceptibility to periodontal disease

Local risk factors (predisposing factors)	Systemic risk factors (modifying factors)
Dental plaque-biofilm retention factors: • Tooth anatomy • Restoration margins • Intra-oral appliances, such as the removal of partial dentures	Age

Oral dryness
• Decreased saliva flow
• Reduced quality of saliva
  • Sjögren's syndrome
  • Medications
  • Mouth-breathing
	Smoking

	Metabolic factors • Hyperglycaemia Nutritional factors • Vitamin C Pharmacological agents Sex hormones • Puberty • Pregnancy Haematological conditions

7 Epidemiology of oral and oropharyngeal cancer

Figure 7.1 Head and neck cancer (C00–C14, C30–C32), European age-standardised incidence rates, UK, 1993–2018.
Source: *Cancer Research UK 2023. Reproduced with permission from Cancer Research UK.*

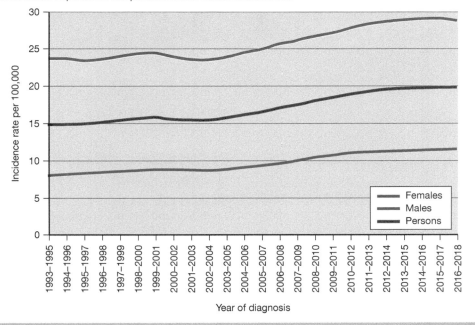

Table 7.2 Risk factors for oral and oropharyngeal cancer

Risk factor	Notes
Smoking tobacco	Oral cancer is three times more common in smokers compared with those who have never smoked.
Smokeless tobacco	Increases the risk of oral cancer between 2 and 7 times.
Betel quid (a combination of betel leaf, areca nut and slaked lime)	Quid increases the risk of oral cancer by 3.5 (used without tobacco) and 7 times (used with tobacco). The use of betel (a type of nut with stimulant properties) is widespread in the Asia and Pacific region and is responsible for the high incidence of oral cancer in those areas. Immigrants from those areas may continue the practice in the United Kingdom, e.g. Bangladeshi women.
Alcohol	Consumption of alcohol increases the risk of oral cancer. It has been calculated that risk increases by 35% in men and 9% in women for every 1.5 units of alcohol consumed per day.
Human papilloma virus (HPV)	HPV, particularly strain 16, is associated with oral cancer and is increasingly accepted as a risk factor. Transmission is by oral sex. An estimated 8% of oral cavity cancers and 14% of oropharyngeal cancers in the United Kingdom are linked to HPV infection. A large US population survey of oral prevalence of HPV infection found an overall 7% population prevalence, with bimodal peaks at 10% in 25–30- and 50–55-year-old males. Risk factors for oral HPV carriage were also identified. These included smoking, alcohol, number of sexual partners, number of oral sex partners, and open-mouth kissing.
Family history	Head and neck cancer risk is 70% higher in people with a family (particularly sibling) history of head and neck cancer versus those without such a history.
Socio-economic status (SES)	There is evidence that oral cancer is associated with SES, even when other risk factors, such as tobacco and alcohol, have been controlled for.
Diet	Malnutrition is particularly associated with excess alcohol consumption and smoking. There is some suggestion that consuming a diet rich in fruits and vegetables, and therefore in antioxidants, protects against oral cancer.

Recording oral cancer

The incidence (risk) burden of cancer in a population is best measured by incidence rates. Cancer incidence rates are the number of new cases diagnosed in the population over a given period of time (usually a year) expressed as a rate by dividing this by the total population at risk during that period (denominator). The denominator is usually adjusted to account for different age profiles in different populations referenced to a standard population, which has a known population age structure. This is often the European Standard Population, which is a theoretical population adding up to a total of 100,000 persons. Incidence rate data are available from routinely collected data in cancer registries. Changes in the incidence of all head and neck cancers in the United Kingdom between 1993 and 2018 are shown in Figure 7.1.

Table 7.1 UK Cancer registry data: numbers (N) and (European) age-standardised incidence rates per 100,000 person-years, by sex

Country	Oral cavity cancer Incidence rate	(OCC) N	Oropharyngeal cancer Incidence rate	(OPC) N	Year Date
England					2016
Females	4.8 per 100,000	1309	2.7 per 100,000	712	
Males	7.3 per 100,000	1779	9.1 per 100,000	2265	
Northern Ireland					2016
Females	3.9 per 100,000	34	2.1 per 100,000	18	
Males	5.9 per 100,000	46	6.8 per 100,000	55	
Scotland					2016
Females	5.6 per 100,000	160	2.7 per 100,000	77	
Males	10.0 per 100,000	240	9.7 per 100,000	247	
Wales					2015
Females	3.7 per 100,000	64	2.9 per 100,000	48	
Males	7.4 per 100,000	112	10.5 per 100,000	159	

Source: *UK Cancer Registries.*

Terminology

There is an emerging consensus that cancers affecting the mouth should be differentiated into oropharyngeal cancer and oral cancer. **Oropharyngeal cancer** has been defined using the International Classification of Diseases (ICD) sites as: the base of the tongue (C01), lingual tonsil (C2.4), tonsil (C09), oropharynx (C10), and pharynx unspecified including Waldeyer's ring/overlapping sites of oral cavity and pharynx (C14); while **oral cavity cancer** includes: the inner lip (C00.3–C00.9), other and unspecified parts of the tongue (C02) (excluding lingual tonsil [C2.4]), gum (C03), floor of the mouth (C04), palate (C05), and other and unspecified parts of the mouth (C06).

This differentiation has arisen primarily due to differences in proposed aetiology at different sites and different age groups affected.

The incidence of oral and oropharyngeal cancer – United Kingdom

Oral cancer

In 2016, 3744 people in the UK were diagnosed with oral cancer (Table 7.1). The risk of oral cancer increases with age. Age-standardised incidence rates of mouth cancer are higher in Scotland than the rest of the UK and are rising in England and Wales. Mouth cancer is much more common among males than females, with a ratio of approximately 2:1; it is more common among older age groups, with the peak age for diagnosis being 66–70 years.

Data from Scotland reveal wide socio-economic inequalities in the incidence of oral cancer, with those from the lowest socioeconomic groups having a nearly threefold greater incidence risk ratio than those from the highest socioeconomic groups, while data from London suggests some South East Asian ethnic groups have higher incidence rate ratios of mouth cancer than their white counterparts.

Oropharyngeal cancer

Oropharyngeal cancer incidence rates are rising rapidly in all four countries in the United Kingdom, with 2977 people in England diagnosed with oropharyngeal cancer in 2016. In Wales, oropharyngeal cancer in men now exceeds oral cavity cancer rates (Table 7.1) and has been reported as the fastest-rising incidence of any cancer in Scotland. The risk of oropharyngeal cancer is more than three times higher among men than women and over three-fold higher among those from more deprived socio-economic areas than less deprived areas. There is some evidence that people with human papillomavirus (HPV)-related cancers (such as oropharyngeal cancer) are diagnosed at a younger age. However, this is not substantially younger than oral cavity cancer, with the peak age for oropharyngeal cancer diagnosis being 61–65 years.

Mortality and survival

There are no UK-wide statistics available for mouth and oropharyngeal cancer survival by stage. Outcomes are influenced by site and particularly stage of the cancer at diagnosis. The disease is more prevalent in those from lower socioeconomic backgrounds who are often not in regular contact with medical and dental services. The disease is often relatively painless in its early stages, and patients can be unaware or fail to seek help until the cancer is at a relatively advanced stage.

Data from the United States of America (USA) suggest that more than 75 out of 100 people survive their oral cancer for one year or more after they are diagnosed, and around 55 out of 100 people survive for five years or more. In the case of oropharyngeal cancer, almost 80 out of 100 survive their cancer for a year or more after diagnosis, and 60 out of 100 survive for five years or more after diagnosis.

The incidence of oral cancer – International

The incidence of oral cancer varies around the world. In Europe, oral cancer accounts for about 2% of all cancers, similar to the United Kingdom. It is highest in Hungary and lowest in Greece. In the USA, oral cancer also accounts for about 2–3% of all cancers. This contrasts with the Indian subcontinent, where oral cancer ranks amongst the three most common types of all cancers. Globally the highest age-standardised incidence rates (per 100,000 person-years) for oral cavity cancer are found in Melanesia, namely Papua New Guinea (males = 22.2; females = 11.9) and South Central Asia (males = 13.3; females = 4.6).

Risk factors for oral cancer

Risk factors for oral cancer are largely attributable to lifestyle factors and are summarised in Table 7.2.

Impact of socio-economic status

The chance of developing oral cancer is greater for those from a low social and economic status (SES). A systematic review and meta-analysis of case-control studies from around the world reported that when compared with individuals from high SES, those with a low occupation-related social class were 2.4 times more likely to develop oral cancer.

Epidemiology of malocclusion, non-carious tooth surface loss and traumatic dental injuries

8

Figure 8.1 **The percentage of adults in the UK with any moderate or severe tooth wear.** Source: *Data from Health and Social Care Information Centre (2011).*

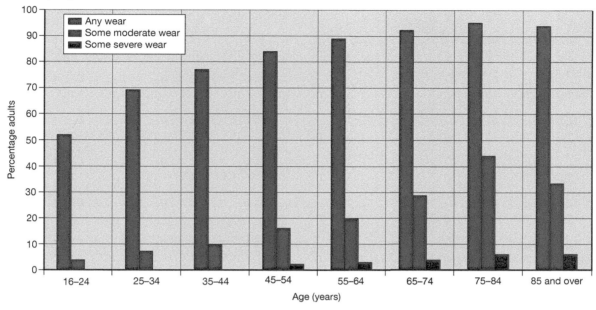

Table 8.1 The modified IOTN as used in dental epidemiological studies

M – Missing teeth	Hypodontia requiring pre-restorative orthodontics or orthodontic space closure to obviate the need for a prosthesis Impeded eruption of teeth Presence of supernumerary teeth Retained deciduous teeth
O – Overjet	Increased overjet greater than 6 mm Reverse overjet greater than 3.5 mm with no masticatory or speech difficulties Reverse overjet greater than 1 mm but less than 3.5 mm with recorded masticatory and speech difficulties
C – Crossbites	Anterior or posterior crossbites with greater than 2 mm discrepancy between retruded contact position and intercuspal position
D – Displacement of contact points (crowding)	Contact point displacements greater than 4 mm
O – Overbite	Lateral or anterior open bites greater than 4 mm Deep overbite with gingival or palatal trauma

If any one of the above occlusal anomalies is present, the subject is said to have a definite need for orthodontic treatment.
Source: *Adapted from Burden et al. (2001).*

Table 8.2 Orthodontic condition of 12- and 15-year-old children in England, Wales and Northern Ireland, 2013

			Percentages
	12 years	15 years	Total
Children undergoing orthodontic treatment at the time of the survey	9	18	13
Children not undergoing orthodontic treatment at the time of the survey			
Unmet orthodontic treatment need (dental health component)	36	20	28
Unmet orthodontic treatment need (aesthetic component Score 8–10)	10	5	7
Any unmet orthodontic treatment need (dental health component or aesthetic component Score 8–10)	37	20	28

Source: *NHS Digital (2015).*

Dental Public Health at a Glance, Second Edition. Ivor G. Chestnutt.
© 2024 John Wiley & Sons Ltd. Published 2024 by John Wiley & Sons Ltd.

Malocclusion

Malocclusion describes the situation where the interdigitation and alignment of the teeth and jaws are less than ideal. This occurs due to misalignment of the teeth, or a discrepancy in the underlying relationship of the skeletal base or a combination of both. Clinically, malocclusion is measured using the **Index of Orthodontic Treatment Need (IOTN)**. The index has two parts: a dental health component (DHC) and an aesthetic component (AC). The DHC is graded 1–5, where 1 = no treatment need and 5 = definite treatment need. The AC comprises a series of 10 intraoral clinical photographs in which the attractiveness of the teeth decreases from 1 to 10. The measurements required to undertake a full IOTN assessment are too time-consuming for application in epidemiological surveys, so a modified version of the IOTN has been developed – this uses a simpler DHC plus the original AC.

The modified version of the IOTN examines five aspects of dentition: Missing teeth, overjet, crossbites, displacement of contact points (crowding) and overbite, remembered using the acronym MOCDO (Table 8.1).

The orthodontic condition of 12- and 15-year-old children in England, Wales and Northern Ireland, as recorded in the 2013 Children's Dental Health Survey, is shown in Table 8.2.

Qualification for treatment by the National Health Service

In the United Kingdom, the IOTN is used by the National Health Service to determine whether a patient's malocclusion is sufficiently severe to merit treatment. To qualify, the DHC must be three or greater or the AC must be six or greater.

Non-carious tooth surface loss (tooth wear)

Tooth surface loss (TSL) can result from erosion, attrition or abrasion. Erosion results from the action of acidic foods and drinks (e.g. carbonated beverages) or the acidic contents of the stomach after repeated vomiting (as occurs in some eating disorders) or gastric regurgitation. Attrition results from the contact of teeth with the opposing dentition and abrasion from the contact of teeth with external objects placed in the mouth, such as hard toothbrushes and abrasive toothpaste.

Tooth surface loss in children

A degree of attrition in the primary dentition is normal. However, exposure to a diet high in acidic foods and especially carbonated drinks has resulted in concerns over the degree of tooth wear in teenagers. In the 2013 Children's Dental Health Survey, tooth surface loss (TSL) was measured on the upper incisors and molar teeth. The prevalence of TSL at age 15 by various factors is shown in Table 8.3.

Tooth surface loss in adults

Tooth wear was measured in the 2009 Adult Dental Health Survey. In those adults with teeth, 77% showed some degree of tooth wear, 15% had moderate wear, and 2% exhibited severe tooth loss. As would be expected, tooth wear and the severity of tooth wear increased with age, as shown in Figure 8.1. A greater proportion of males (82%) experienced tooth wear than females (73%).

Traumatic dental injuries

Accidental injury to children's teeth is common. The frequency of injury is greater in boys, in children with an increased overjet and children from households from a lower social and economic class.

Estimates of the prevalence of accidental damage vary across surveys due to differences in the definitions of injury. A 2018 systematic review estimated the global prevalence of traumatic dental injuries to be 21% for primary and 15% for permanent teeth.

Prevention of traumatic dental injuries

Preventing traumatic dental injuries has focussed on providing mouthguards when participating in contact sports. While this seems a sensible measure intuitively, the degree to which mouthguards prevent dental injury has yet to be definitively established. The main limitation of this approach is that the majority of traumatic dental injuries do not occur when participating in organised sports but as a result of accidents during normal play and during slips, trips and falls. Dental injuries as a result of cycling, skateboarding and riding scooters are also regularly encountered in emergency dental clinics. Preventive strategies need to focus on increasing public awareness of dental injuries and, in particular, what to do in the event of an injury.

Table 8.3 Percentage of 15-year-old with tooth surface loss in two or more permanent incisors or four teeth overall in England, Wales and Northern Ireland, 2013

By country	England	Wales	Northern Ireland	Total
Surface loss into dentine in at least two permanent incisors	3	4	4	3
Surface loss into dentine in at least four permanent incisors or molars	3	1	3	3
Either of these	4	4	4	4

By sex	Male	Female
Surface loss into dentine in at least two permanent incisors	3	3
Surface loss into dentine in at least four permanent incisors or molars	2	3
Either of these	4	4

By eligibility for free school meals (as a proxy for social and economic status)	Eligible	Not eligible
Surface loss into dentine in at least two permanent incisors	5	3
Surface loss into dentine in at least four permanent incisors or molars	7	2
Either of these	8	3

By frequency of drinking sugary drinks	<1 per day	1–3 times per day	4 or more times per day
Surface loss into dentine in at least two permanent incisors	2	4	5
Surface loss into dentine in at least four permanent incisors or molars	1	3	4
Either of these	2	4	5

Source: *NHS Digital (2015).*

⑨ National trends in oral health

Figure 9.1   Loss of all natural teeth by age in UK 1968–2009. Source: *Data from Health and Social Care Information Centre (2011). (2009 = England, Wales & N Ireland only)*

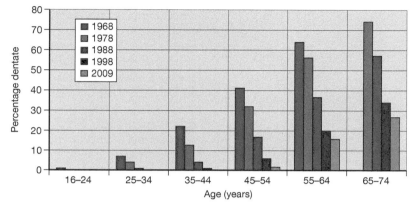

Figure 9.2   Time series and future projection of adult oral health in the UK 1998–2030. Source: *NHS England Digital Analytical Team (2014).*

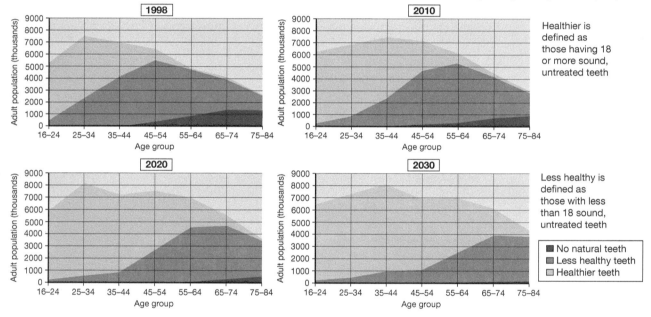

Healthier is defined as those having 18 or more sound, untreated teeth

Less healthy is defined as those with less than 18 sound, untreated teeth

- No natural teeth
- Less healthy teeth
- Healthier teeth

Figure 9.3   A schematic of the changing picture of oral health in the U.K

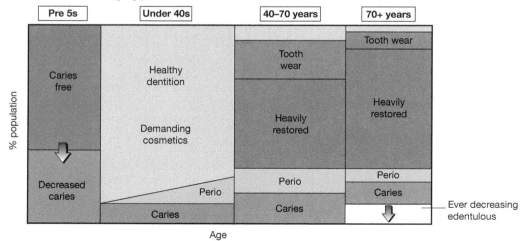

Dental Public Health at a Glance, Second Edition. Ivor G. Chestnutt.
© 2024 John Wiley & Sons Ltd. Published 2024 by John Wiley & Sons Ltd.

The decennial adult oral health surveys (Chapter 5) provide data that show how oral health has changed in the past four decades. It is possible to model how these changes will be carried forward in time and infer how future oral health and oral care needs will change.

Changes in oral health

Decrease in tooth loss

The most remarkable change in oral health over the last century has been a dramatic reduction in the proportion of the adult population who have had all of their teeth extracted. In the mid-twentieth century, it was common for people in the United Kingdom to have all their teeth extracted in early adulthood. This procedure was known as a 'dental clearance'. In the 1968 Adult Dental Health Survey, edentulous patients (i.e. those who had had all of their teeth extracted) were asked how many teeth were removed at the time they were rendered edentulous. In response, two-thirds said that they had had 12 or more teeth removed, and one-third had had 21 or more teeth removed – a scenario that is difficult to imagine today. Tooth removal was often carried out under general anaesthesia in dental practices. This reflected attitudes to oral health at that time, where removal of teeth and provision of complete dentures were often the only solutions to the high levels of dental caries that were prevalent.

Since the late 1960s, the proportion of the population who have lost all of their own teeth has fallen dramatically (Figure 9.1), and overall, the proportion of the UK population who are edentulous fell from 30% in 1978 to 6% in 2009. Whilst an Adult Dental Health Survey was conducted in England in 2021, this did not include an oral examination; hence, the latest comparable data available is from 2009.

Increase in sound and untreated teeth

Figure 9.2 shows a projection of how the proportion of the population with 18 or more sound untreated teeth will have changed between 1998 and 2030.

Changes in oral health across the generations

A schematic picture of what is happening to oral health across the generations is shown in Figure 9.3. While dental caries remains a problem in children from disadvantaged backgrounds (Chapter 19), oral health in children and young adults has improved dramatically (Figure 5.4).

A key factor in improving oral health in the United Kingdom has been the introduction of fluoride-containing toothpaste. Fluoride toothpaste has been widely available since the early 1970s and is the factor that is often quoted as the key determinant of improved oral health in the last half-century.

People in middle to early older age, born prior to the general availability of fluoride toothpaste, often have retained the majority of their teeth because they have been able to take advantage of the increased availability and technical capability of dental services. Many of their teeth are heavily restored and will require continuing maintenance into old age. This segment of the population has been referred to as the 'heavy metal generation', – perhaps reflecting their musical tastes, but also that their dentition is largely composed of metal restorations.

The proportion of older people who are edentulous will decrease over time so by 2030, the proportion of the population who will have lost all of their teeth will be very small (Figure 9.2).

Reasons for improved oral health

The following are the likely reasons for the improvements seen in oral health:

- Introduction and widespread availability of fluoride toothpaste.
- Changed public and professional attitudes to tooth loss.
- Increased access to dental care.
- Development of dental technology, especially in relation to endodontics, crown and bridge techniques and implants.

Implications of changes in oral health

The changes described have implications for both clinicians and commissioners of oral care.

Implications for clinicians

- Younger patients with essentially healthy dentitions may increasingly demand cosmetic and aesthetic treatments.
- Toothwear will increase, and dentists will need to manage an increasing number of patients with worn dentition (Figure 8.1).
- Increased tooth retention in association with gingival recession heightens the likelihood of root caries development.
- With age, the degree of periodontal attachment loss increases, so the proportion of older people with periodontal problems will increase.
- Most old people will in future have teeth, and in the majority of cases, a good number of teeth. The number of old people in the population is increasing as the baby boomers born in the period 1946–1964 become the aged population. People are living longer, so there will be more old people to treat, and nearly all of them will have teeth.
- If patients eventually lose all of their teeth at an older age, adaptation to dentures can be a problem due to reduced muscle balance.
- Older people are likely to have co-morbidities that either affect their oral health or complicate the provision of oral care.
- In the past, performing simple extractions or constructing dentures in a domiciliary setting was relatively easy. It is more challenging to treat an older person who may have lost mental capacity due to dementia and who has toothache associated with a heavily restored dentition.

Implications for commissioners

- Oral health promotion needs for older dentate adults have to be considered, e.g. addressing changing diets on retirement.
- Skill-mix issues.
- Use of hygienists and therapists to treat low-need younger people.
- Target dentists' skills at more high-need older people.
- Training needs of future dental professionals may change, e.g. less frequent construction of complete dentures.
- The requirement to commission access to care for people in nursing and residential care homes.

International oral health

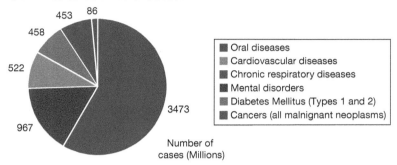

Figure 10.1 Comparison of estimated global case numbers for selected non-communicable diseases. Source: *Adapted and reproduced with permission from the World Health Organisation: Global oral health status report: towards universal health coverage for oral health by 2030. Geneva: World Health Organisation; 2022. Licence: CC BY-NC-SA 3.0 IGO.*

Legend:
- Oral diseases
- Cardiovascular diseases
- Chronic respiratory diseases
- Mental disorders
- Diabetes Mellitus (Types 1 and 2)
- Cancers (all malnignant neoplasms)

Number of cases (Millions)

Data are for all ages and both sexes from Global Burden of Diseases 2019; oral diseases do not include lip and oral cavity cancer. A standard method has been applied to incorporate the latest UN population estimates.

Figure 10.2 Estimated cases and prevalence of severe periodontal disease* per WHO region.

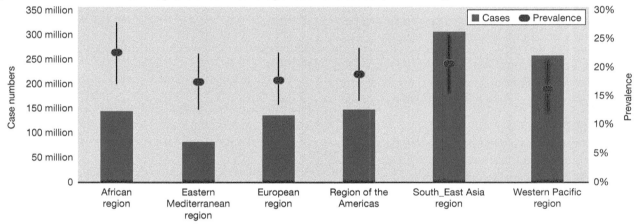

*Severe disease defined as at least one pocket > 6 mm. Data are for ages greater than five years, both sexes, from Global Burden of Disease 2019.

The World Health Organization and oral health

Previous chapters have looked at oral health in the United Kingdom. However, it is important to understand the epidemiology of oral disease across the world. The body responsible for securing an oversight of global oral health status is the World Health Organisation (WHO). At the 74th World Health Assembly in 2021, the WHO approved a 'Resolution on Oral Health'. The Resolution recommends a shift from the traditional curative approach towards a preventive approach that includes the promotion of oral health within the family, schools and workplaces, and includes timely, comprehensive and inclusive care within the primary health-care system.

Resource allocation is a key issue in promoting oral health and securing access to dental care. In developing countries, getting oral health onto the agenda can be a problem when other health issues may be seen as more pressing. Recognition of the common risk factor approach (Chapter 21) to improving oral health allows oral disease prevention to be incorporated into wider health-promotion activities. The WHO resolution affirms that oral health should be included in the agenda for tackling non-communicable diseases and in universal health coverage programmes.

Global oral health status

A 2022 report issued by the WHO estimated that oral disease affected almost 3.5 billion people in 2019, with three out of four people affected living in middle-income countries. Among the major oral diseases, untreated caries of permanent teeth is the most prevalent, with around 2 billion cases; severe periodontal disease follows with around 1 billion cases, then untreated caries of deciduous teeth with about 510 million cases and edentulism (loss of all teeth) with 350 million cases. The WHO estimates that the combined estimated number of cases of oral diseases globally is about 1 billion higher than cases of all five main non-communicable diseases (mental disorders, cardiovascular disease, diabetes mellitus, chronic respiratory diseases and cancers) combined (Figure 10.1).

Oral disease – International perspective

Across the world, dental caries and periodontal disease are the major contributors to oral ill health.

Dental caries

The estimated global prevalence of dental caries is shown in Tables 10.1 primary and 10.2 permanent teeth, with 42.7% and 28.7% of the population affected, respectively. Between 1990 and 2019, the number of people with caries in their permanent dentition increased by about 640 million, despite a slight decrease in overall prevalence (−2.6%). This significant increase in caries burden is mainly driven by the rise in case numbers due to the population growth in low- and lower-middle-income countries, where prevalence increases of 121% and 74%, respectively, were reported.

Periodontal disease

Severe periodontal disease, defined as the presence of a periodontal pocket of at least 6 mm, is widespread, with a global prevalence of about 19% in adults. This equates to more than one billion cases worldwide. The prevalence and number of cases by WHO region are shown in Figure 10.2.

Oral cancer

The prevalence of oral cancer varies markedly around the world, and overall is the eighth most common cancer. In the United States of America, the prevalence is estimated to be 2.5 cases per 100,000 inhabitants. The highest rates of oral cancer are seen in south-central Asia, where oral cancer is among the three most common types of cancer. This is largely attributed to the widespread habit of using betel and other smokeless tobacco products.

Noma (cancrum oris)

Noma is a disfiguring gangrenous condition that is seen most commonly in sub-Saharan Africa. The prevalence is estimated at 1–7 cases per 1000 population. It predominantly affects children and young people (2–16 years). The disease results in the destruction of the soft tissues of the face and the underlying bone. Risk factors are poverty, malnutrition, poor oral hygiene, residential proximity to livestock and infectious diseases such as measles and herpes viruses. The resulting impaired immune system is thought to allow bacteria such as Fusobacterium necrophorum and Prevotella intermedia to destroy the facial tissues. Acute necrotising gingivitis or ulcers arising from herpes virus infections may initiate the noma lesion. Untreated, 70–90% of patients will die.

HIV/AIDS and oral health

The WHO estimates that at the end of 2021, 38.4 million people around the world were living with the human immunodeficiency virus (HIV). Infection with HIV predisposes the individual to oral infections due to weakened immune defence mechanisms. Common problems faced by individuals with HIV/Aids are xerostomia, candida (thrush), herpes simplex virus-1, herpes zoster, oral hairy leukoplakia and oral warts due to human papillomavirus, Kaposi's sarcoma and aphthous ulcers. Advances in antiretroviral therapy mean that if they are diagnosed promptly, people infected with HIV can expect a near-normal lifespan. This therapy has made some oral problems less common.

Universal health coverage

This term means access to a full range of quality health services when needed, without financial hardship. The WHO has set out a vision of Universal health coverage for oral health for all individuals and communities by 2030 – an ambitious target.

Table 10.1 Estimated prevalence and number of cases of dental caries in *primary* teeth in 2019 and their percentage change from 1990 to 2019 per WHO region

WHO region	Prevalence (2019)	Cases (2019) (Millions)	Percentage change in prevalence (1990–2019)	Percentage change in cases (1990–2019)
African region	38.61%	111.0	−3.40%	87.19%
Eastern Mediterranean region	45.10%	66.4	0.60%	44.35%
European region	39.64%	40.9	−7.22%	−22.10%
Region of the Americas	43.21%	57.5	−2.21%	−2.29%
South-East Asia region	43.77%	135.3	−1.96%	−3.25%
Western Pacific region	46.20%	102.1	−0.20%	−22.75%
GLOBAL	42.71%	5123.8	−3.33%	5.56%

Data are for children aged one to nine years, both sexes, from the Global Database of Disease (2019) and the United Nations Department of Economic and Social Affairs (2019). Source: Reproduced with permission from WHO: Global oral health status report (2022).

Table 10.2 Estimated prevalence and number of cases of dental caries in *permanent* teeth in 2019 and the percentage change of prevalence, cases and population from 1990 to 2019 per WHO region

WHO region	Prevalence (2019)	Cases (2019) (Millions)	Percentage change in prevalence (1990–2019)	Percentage change in cases (1990–2019)	Percentage change in population (1990–2019)
African region	28.50%	262.6	−1.66%	119.94%	114.98%
Eastern Mediterranean region	32.25%	202.2	−0.27%	102.94%	93.08%
European region	33.63%	239.9	−3.91%	6.09%	9.94%
Region of the Americas	28.24%	264.5	−0.05%	46.35%	40.70%
South-East Asia region	28.69%	525.7	0.67%	65.26%	52.38%
Western Pacific region	25.41%	463.9	−6.50%	20.37%	24.96%
GLOBAL	28.70%	2019.7	−2.59%	46.07%	44.79%

Data are for all ages greater than five years, both sexes, from the Global Database of Disease (2019) and the United Nations Department of Economic and Social Affairs (2019). Source: Reproduced with permission from WHO: Global oral health status report (2022).

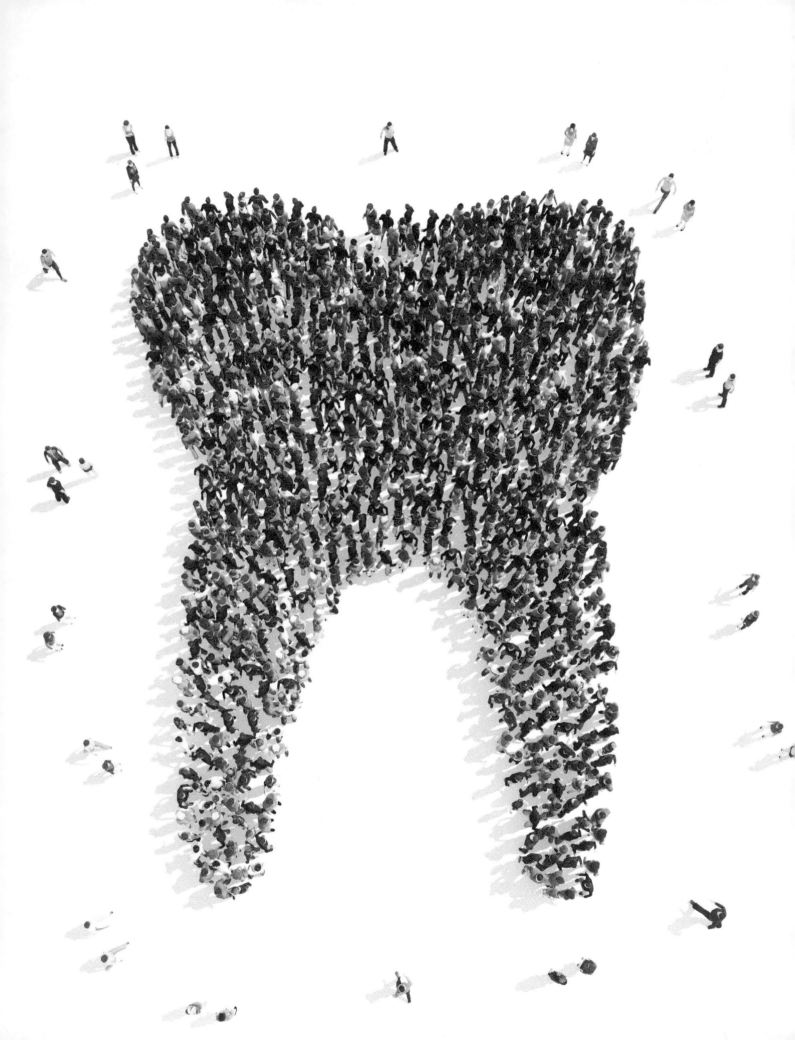

Evidence based dentistry

Part 3

Chapters

Study design

Figure 11.1 Study design in the research process

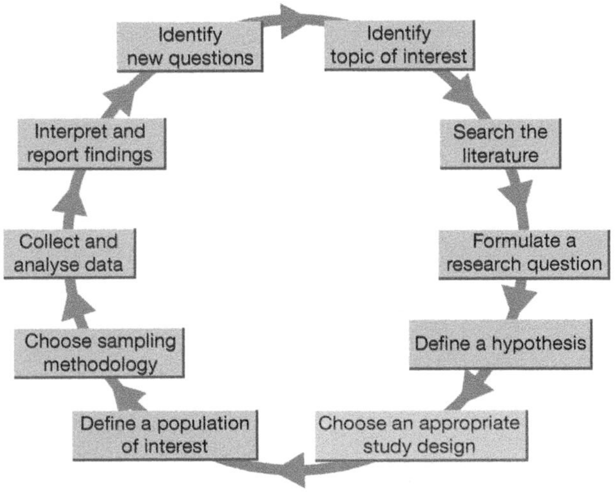

Identify topic of interest → Search the literature → Formulate a research question → Define a hypothesis → Choose an appropriate study design → Define a population of interest → Choose sampling methodology → Collect and analyse data → Interpret and report findings → Identify new questions → Identify topic of interest

Figure 11.2 Observational/Interventional studies

Observational	Interventional
Descriptive Cross-sectional Case-control Cohort	Randomised controlled trial

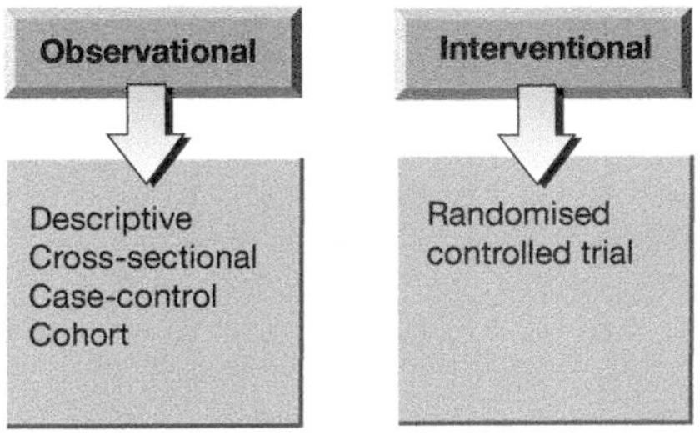

Figure 11.3 Time and study design

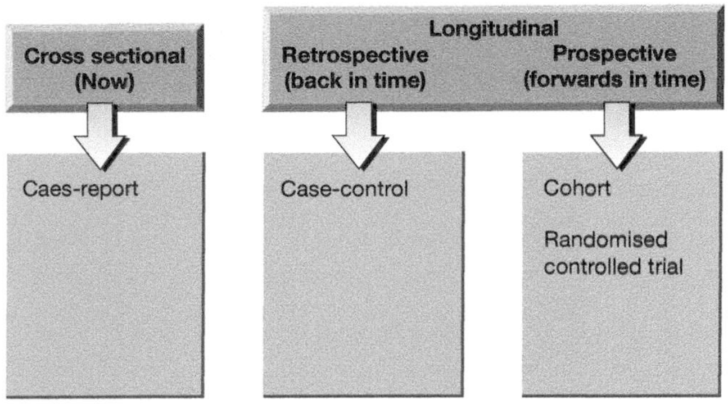

Cross sectional (Now)	Longitudinal	
	Retrospective (back in time)	Prospective (forwards in time)
Caes-report	Case-control	Cohort Randomised controlled trial

Figure 11.4 Primary and secondary studies

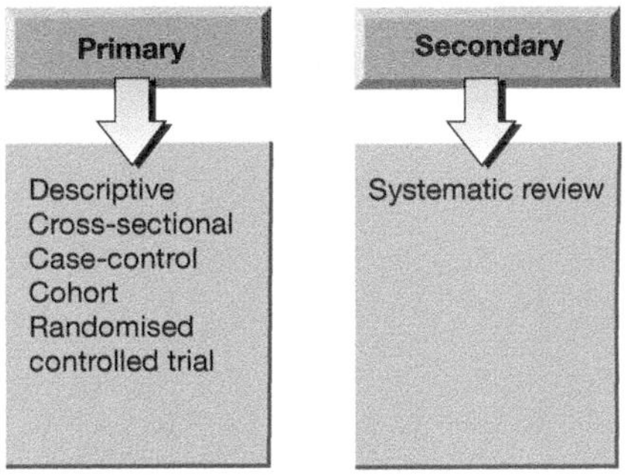

Primary	Secondary
Descriptive Cross-sectional Case-control Cohort Randomised controlled trial	Systematic review

Study design

Study design requires an understanding of the different approaches that may be taken to answer a research question. How the study design fits into the research process is shown in Figure 11.1. Different research questions require different types of study design. The most significant difference between different types of study is the degree to which they control for outside factors such as bias and confounding. A good understanding of study design is fundamental to good research and critical appraisal skills. The principal types of study design are shown in Table 11.1.

Observational and interventional studies

Studies can be described as observational or interventional (Figure 11.2). In observational studies, no attempt is made to alter or interfere with the participants or the environment – as the name suggests, the study is confined to recording facts purely by observation. In interventional studies, the researchers manipulate the participants or their environment in some way – they conduct an experiment.

Time and study design

The time period over which a study is conducted is another fundamental issue in study design. Studies can be described as cross-sectional, so carried out at a point in time. Longitudinal studies follow participants over time, either by looking backward from the present time (retrospective) or looking forward (prospective) (Figure 11.3). The issue of time is crucial, as cause and effect can only be inferred from longitudinal studies.

Dental Public Health at a Glance, Second Edition. Ivor G. Chestnut.
© 2024 John Wiley & Sons Ltd. Published 2024 by John Wiley & Sons Ltd.

Primary and secondary research

Studies can be further categorised as primary or secondary research (Figure 11.4). In primary research, new data are gathered from or about participants or their environment. Secondary research involves the generation of new data from existing studies. The generation of evidence by combining results from different studies (as occurs in a systematic review) is secondary research.

While systematic reviews followed by a meta-analysis (Chapter 18) are the most valued type of secondary research, other review types exist (Table 11.2).

Cause, effect and association

It is crucial to remember that just because two factors are shown to be associated in a study, it does not mean that one necessarily causes the other or vice versa. The following factors, described by Bradford-Hill, can be used to infer that a relationship is causal. As an example, the relationship between cigarette smoking and periodontal attachment loss is used in this way.

Dose-response

A relationship is more likely to be causal if the extent of the disease is linked to the degree of exposure to the causative factor. Periodontal attachment loss is worse in heavy smokers than light smokers, who, in turn, have more attachment loss than nonsmokers.

Change in risk factor

Removal of the suspected causative factor should lead to a reduction in the disease or at least no further progression. Former smokers have less periodontal disease than those who continue to smoke.

Temporal relationship

A causal relationship is more likely if the disease occurs after exposure to the suspected risk factor. This is difficult to demonstrate using the example of periodontal disease and tobacco smoking, but could be shown in a cohort study.

Consistency

A causal relationship is more likely if the relationship between the disease and the suspected causative factor has been shown to hold true in multiple studies. So, in the example of periodontal disease and smoking, studies conducted in different sites around the world have demonstrated that periodontal disease is worse in smokers.

Specificity

In a causal relationship, a postulated causal factor should lead to the disease in question and no other. This is not the case in the example of cigarette smoking, which is causally related to many diseases and conditions other than periodontal disease.

Biological plausibility

Suppose a biological mechanism can be proposed for the suspected causal factor that strengthens the likelihood of a causal relationship. It has been shown that nicotine has vasoconstrictive effects on gingival blood vessels and has detrimental effects on neutrophils. These have been postulated as mechanisms whereby smoking interferes with the host's defence mechanisms, thereby predisposing to periodontal attachment loss.

Experiment

It is possible to demonstrate a causal relationship by experiment – that is the basis of a randomised controlled trial (Chapters 15 and 16). However, this can only be done where the action is to prevent disease or to remove a suspected causative factor. In the smoking and periodontal disease example, it would be possible (although practically difficult) to conduct an experiment to examine the effects of stopping smoking on periodontal health. It would, of course, be unethical to look at the relationship in reverse; that is, to encourage people to smoke in order to examine the effects of smoking tobacco on the periodontal tissues.

Table 11.1 Types of study design

Type of study	
Case report (descriptive) Cross-sectional Case-control Cohort Randomised controlled trial Systematic review	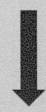 More robust study design More controlled for bias and confounding factors as progress down this list of designs

Table 11.2 Common types of reviews of scientific literature and other reports

Narrative review	The traditional type of literature review, unstructured, does not contain specific inclusion/exclusion criteria, which is good for identifying gaps in the literature but may be subject to bias.
Rapid review	Rapid reviews are undertaken to help support time-sensitive decision-making. Standard systematic review procedures are adapted by removing or modifying some steps.
Scoping review	Designed to identify what material/research there is on a particular topic. Is structured in format, but there are no restrictions on study type/study outcome(s) specified in advance. Can be carried out before embarking on a formal systematic review with more narrowly defined study designs/outcomes or to identify that there is insufficient evidence/no evidence available for a formal systematic review.
Systematic review	Formal and structured, they have a very specific focus (See Chapter 17).
Umbrella review	Also termed 'a review of reviews' – find, contrast and synthesise the findings from other systematic-style reviews.

Case reports and cross-sectional studies

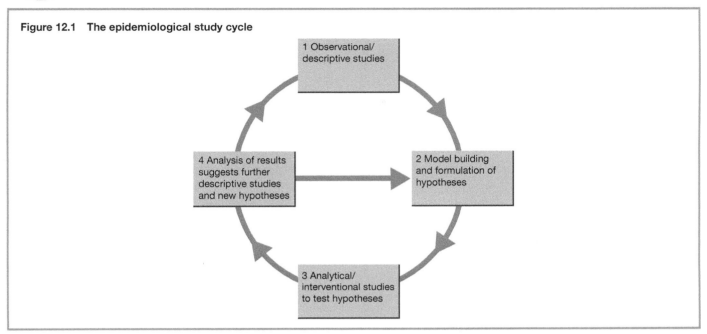

Figure 12.1 The epidemiological study cycle

1 Observational/descriptive studies

2 Model building and formulation of hypotheses

3 Analytical/interventional studies to test hypotheses

4 Analysis of results suggests further descriptive studies and new hypotheses

Case reports

The simplest type of research report, a case report, is a description of a single case or series of cases, typically of an unusual finding or alternative means of managing a condition. It is often accompanied by a brief literature review that describes similar cases reported previously and a discussion of the implications of the case or cases reported.

Advantages of case reports

- Useful for describing unusual events or rarely encountered situations.
- Educational – may help those who subsequently encounter a similar case.

- Maybe the first report of a never before recognised condition – for example, hairy leukoplakia, one of the oral manifestations of Acquired Immune Deficiency Syndrome (AIDS), was initially reported in a series of case reports.

Disadvantages of case reports

- They are reports of only one or a few cases and are anecdotal and subjective in nature.
- There is no control for bias and confounding.
- They cannot be used to conclude the cause, prevention or definitive management of the condition described.

Dental Public Health at a Glance, Second Edition. Ivor G. Chestnutt.
© 2024 John Wiley & Sons Ltd. Published 2024 by John Wiley & Sons Ltd.

Cross-sectional studies (surveys)

Cross-sectional studies or surveys are commonly used in dental public health. They can be used to:

- Estimate the prevalence of a disease/condition/habit
- Report the current health status of a defined group
- Establish reference ranges
- Determine the cut-off points for a diagnostic test.

The most common form of cross-sectional survey is the series of epidemiological surveys that are carried out to determine the oral health status of a representative sample of the population. In the United Kingdom, there have been two major series of surveys.

Decennial surveys of child and adult oral health

These surveys were commissioned by the Departments of Health in the United Kingdom.

The child surveys were conducted in 1973, 1983, 1993, 2003 and 2013. The adult surveys were conducted in 1968 (England and Wales only), 1978, 1988, 1998 and 2009. In the past, these studies have covered all constituent countries of the United Kingdom.

However, following the devolution of responsibility for the National Health Service to the administrations in Belfast, Cardiff and Edinburgh, increasingly oral health surveys are being conducted by individual nations according to their perceived needs, and the very useful pan-UK aspect of the surveys are being lost.

British Association for the Study of Community Dentistry surveys

Since 1986, a series of surveys, focusing mainly on children but more recently including limited surveys of specific adult groups, have been undertaken by the Community/Salaried Dental Services. These studies are commissioned by local health bodies (Health Boards in Scotland and Wales, Local Authorities in England). The criteria for these surveys have been drawn up by the British Association for the Study of Community Dentistry. They are designed to guide the sampling procedure and criteria used to record the clinical conditions being measured – primarily dental caries.

International oral health surveys

In the United States, the National Health and Nutrition Examination Survey (NHANES) comprises a series of interviews and physical examinations of a representative sample of the US population. This includes oral health. The programme has been running since the 1960s.

The World Health Organization (WHO) has produced a manual to guide the conduct of oral health surveys. The idea is to provide a standard that, if followed, will allow comparison across countries. The WHO maintains a database of international oral health surveys.

The Global Burden of Disease Study (GBD) is a systematic, scientific effort to quantify the magnitude of all major diseases, risk factors and intermediate clinical outcomes in a highly standardised way, to allow for comparisons over time, across populations and between health problems.

The Global Oral Health Status Report uses the latest available data from the GBD project, the International Agency for Research on Cancer (IARC) and global WHO surveys. The report is directed at policymakers, practitioners, researchers, development agencies and members of the private sector and civil society.

In addition to these series of cross-sectional surveys, one-off surveys, which can take the form of clinical examinations or questionnaires – either administered in person, by telephone, by post or online – can be used to gather data at a given point in time.

Advantages of cross-sectional studies (surveys)

- Can be used to determine how common a condition is – the prevalence (Chapter 3)
- Can be used to determine access to services at a given point in time
- Can be used to gather current opinion (opinion poll)
- Are easy to conduct compared to longitudinal studies.

Disadvantages of cross-sectional studies (surveys)

- As they lack a temporal element, cross-sectional studies cannot be used to make causal inferences.

Trend data

From a series of cross-sectional surveys, it is possible to determine trends. For example, from the Adult Dental Health Surveys, it has been possible to show that the proportion of the population who are edentulous (have lost all of their teeth) has decreased from 30% in 1978 to 6% in 2009. It should be noted that although trends can be established from a series of cross-sectional studies, this does not equate to disease increment, as different individuals are involved in successive surveys.

Ecological studies

Ecological studies are a form of cross-sectional study, where populations or whole communities form the unit of analysis. Ecological studies often determine cause and effect by comparing geographical areas. Many useful observations have been made from ecological studies, but they are prone to confounding caused by differences in the age and gender structure of the populations being compared. For this reason, the use of standardised data is important (Chapter 3). In dental public health, investigations of the effects of water fluoridation are often in the form of ecological studies.

An important issue is the ecological fallacy. This occurs when conclusions are drawn from groups of individuals and applied to individuals. For example, suppose data are available detailing the prevalence of dental caries in a series of school classes in a town. If we were to visit the class with the highest caries score and select a child from that class and say that he/she had a high caries score, that would be an example of an ecological fallacy. Because the caries level in the class as a whole is high, it does not follow that an individual child picked at random from that class will have a high caries experience. That child could well be one of the few with a low caries score.

The epidemiological study cycle

The epidemiological study cycle demonstrates how observational studies can be used to inform theory and models that can subsequently be investigated using interventional studies (Figure 12.1).

A good example of the epidemiological study cycle is the studies conducted in the United States in the first half of the twentieth century on water fluoridation (Chapter 27). Observational studies of dental fluorosis show that the association between the level of fluoride in the water supply and caries prevalence led to the hypothesis that by adding fluoride to the public water supply, the prevalence of dental caries could be reduced. This theory was tested using an intervention study, and water fluoridation was shown to be an effective means of preventing dental caries (detail in Table 27.1).

13 Case-control studies

Figure 13.1 Case-control and cohort studies

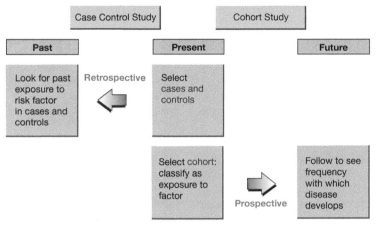

Figure 13.2 Case-control study

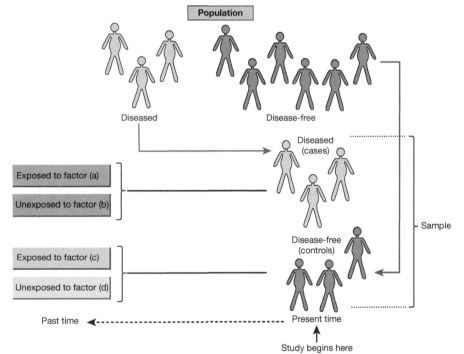

Figure 13.3 Analysis of a case-control study

Reported as an odds ratio

$$\text{Odds ratio} = \frac{\text{Odds of being a case in exposed group}}{\text{Odds of being a case in unexposed group}}$$

	Exposed to factor		
	Yes	No	Total
Disease status			
Case	a	b	a+b
Control	c	d	c+d
Total	a+c	b+d	a+b+c+d

$$\text{Odds}_{exp} = \frac{\left[\dfrac{a}{a+c}\right]}{\left[\dfrac{c}{a+c}\right]} = \frac{a}{c}$$

$$\text{Odds}_{unexp} = \frac{\left[\dfrac{b}{b+d}\right]}{\left[\dfrac{d}{b+d}\right]} = \frac{b}{d}$$

Therefore estimated odds ratio =

$$\frac{a/c}{b/d} = \frac{a \times d}{b \times c}$$

Typically reported as odds ratio and confidence interval of the odds ratio

Dental Public Health at a Glance, Second Edition. Ivor G. Chestnutt.
© 2024 John Wiley & Sons Ltd. Published 2024 by John Wiley & Sons Ltd.

Case-control studies

A case-control study is an observational study design that, at the outset, selects cases (individuals with the disease or condition of interest) and matches these with controls (individuals who do not have the disease or condition of interest). Cases and controls are usually matched for possible confounding factors such as age and gender. This means that the case and control groups will have approximately the same age and gender, so the influence of these parameters is reduced. The researchers then examine the difference in exposure to suspected risk/aetiological factors of both cases and controls. Case-control studies are retrospective in nature (Figure 13.1). They focus on events that have happened at or prior to the selection of the participants.

Analysis of a case-control study

A 2×2 table can be constructed from which the odds of being a case in the exposed group can be compared with the odds of being a case in the unexposed group. An estimated odds ratio can be calculated (Figures 13.2 and 13.3). Odds ratios are usually presented ± the 95% confidence interval (CI). This represents the degree of certainty surrounding the estimated odds ratio. An odds ratio of 1 means that there is no difference in risk between the case and control groups. If the odds ratio is greater than 1 then exposure to the suspected risk factor implies a greater risk of developing the disease/condition being investigated. An odds ratio of less than 1 implies that exposure to the factor under investigation actually reduces the risk of the disease/condition.

Advantages of case-control studies

- Generally relatively quick, cheap and easy to perform
- More than one risk factor can be investigated
- Can be conducted with relatively few cases
- Good for investigating the cause of rare diseases (because it is possible to identify all cases from more than one site)
- No loss to follow-up.

Disadvantages of case-control studies

- Require availability of historical records of exposures. If this has not been recorded or there is bias in recording, it can lead to incorrect assumptions about exposure to the suspected risk factor.
- **Recall bias** occurs when cases have an erroneous memory of exposure to risk factors. They may, for example, put greater emphasis on exposure to a suspected risk factor than do controls, thereby biasing the exposure record
- An adequate control group may be difficult to define or obtain.

Box 13.1 Example of a case-control study

Joint effect of human papillomavirus exposure, smoking and alcohol on risk of oral squamous cell carcinoma.
Yang et al. (2023). *BMC Cancer. 23(1):*

BACKGROUND: Smoking, alcohol consumption, and human papillomavirus (HPV) infection are known risk factors for oral squamous cell carcinoma (OSCC), including SCC of the oro-pharynx (SCCOP) and SCC of the oral cavity (SCCOC). Researchers have examined these risk factors independently, but few have observed the potential risk of their interaction. This study investigated the interactions among these risk factors and the risk of OSCC.

METHODS: A total of 377 patients with newly diagnosed SCCOP and SCCOC and 433 frequency-matched cancer-free controls by age and sex were included. Multivariable logistic regression was performed to calculate ORs and 95% CIs.

RESULTS: We found that overall OSCC risk was independently associated with smoking (adjusted OR(aOR), 1.4; 95%CI, 1.0–2.0), alcohol consumption (aOR, 1.6; 95%CI, 1.1–2.2), and HPV16 seropositivity (aOR, 3.3; 95%CI, 2.2–4.9), respectively. Additionally, we found that HPV16 seropositivity increased the risk of overall OSCC in ever-smokers (aOR, 6.8; 95%CI, 3.4–13.4) and ever-drinkers (aOR, 4.8; 95%CI, 2.9–8.0), while HPV16-seronegative ever-smokers and ever-drinkers had less than a twofold increase in risk of overall OSCC (aORs, 1.2; 95%CI, 0.8–1.7 and 1.8; 95%CI, 1.2–2.7, respectively). Furthermore, the increased risk was particularly high for SCCOP in HPV16-seropositive ever-smokers (aOR, 13.0; 95%CI, 6.0–27.7) and HPV16-seropositive ever-drinkers (aOR, 10.8; 95%CI, 5.8–20.1), while the similar increased risk was not found in SCCOC.

CONCLUSION: These results suggest a strong combined effect of HPV16 exposure, smoking, and alcohol on overall OSCC, which may indicate a strong interaction between HPV16 infection and smoking and alcohol consumption, particularly for SCCOP.

Source: *Yang et al. (2023). Reproduced with permission from BMC/ Springer Nature Group.*

The example in Box 13.1 demonstrates the use of a case-control study to determine the effect of human papillomavirus exposure, smoking and alcohol use on the risk of developing oral squamous cell carcinoma. The results demonstrate that oral squamous cell carcinoma was independently associated with smoking, drinking alcohol and evidence of past exposure to human papillomavirus, with adjusted Odds Ratios of 1.4, 1.6 and 3.3, respectively. The study also demonstrates the additional risk associated with more than one investigated risk factors. So, for example, those who had evidence of human papillomavirus exposure and who also smoked increased their odds of developing oral cancer to 6.8. The odds associated with developing cancer in the oro-pharynx were particularly associated with HPV16 infection – the adjusted odds ratio being 13.0 for those who had past exposure and who also smoked tobacco.

14 Cohort studies

Figure 14.1 Cohort study

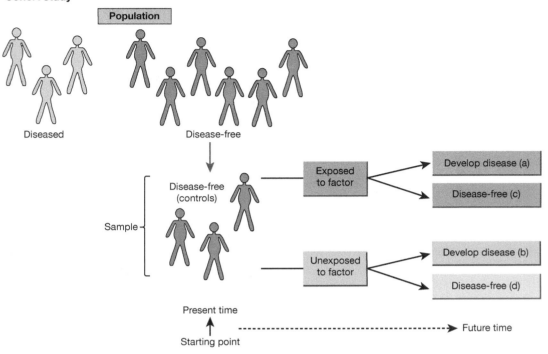

Figure 14.2 Analysis of a cohort study

Because patients are followed can determine risk (compare: estimated odds in case/control studies)

Estimated risk of disease in the exposed group

$risk_{exp} = a/(a+c)$

Estimated risk of disease in the unexposed group

$risk_{unexp} = b/(b+d)$

Estimated relative risk

$= risk_{exp}/risk_{unexp}$

$$= \frac{a/(a+c)}{b/(b+d)}$$

Results are expressed as relative risk plus confidence intervals

	Exposed to factor		
	Yes	No	Total
Disease status			
Yes	a	b	a+b
No	c	d	c+d
Total	a+c	b+d	a+b+c+d

Dental Public Health at a Glance, Second Edition. Ivor G. Chestnutt.

Cohort studies

A cohort study is a form of observational study in which the participants are followed over a period of time from the starting point. A cohort study is prospective in nature. That is, participants are followed over time (Figures 13.1 and 14.1). At the beginning of the study, the participants are free of the disease/condition of interest, but vary in their exposure to possible risk factors. Over time, they are examined and separated into those who do and those who do not develop the condition of interest. The differences in exposure to risk factors are observed, and the relative risk of developing the disease can be calculated depending on exposure to the examined risk factors.

Analysis of a cohort study

A 2×2 table can be constructed from which it is possible to calculate the estimated risk of developing the disease in those exposed to the risk factor. The estimated risk of developing the disease can also be calculated in those unexposed to the risk factor. The relative risk can, therefore, be calculated as the risk in the exposed group divided by the risk in the unexposed group (Figure 14.2). This is usually presented along with the 95% confidence intervals, which estimate the degree of precision of the estimated relative risk.

Advantages of cohort studies

- The time sequence of exposure to the suspected risk factor and development of the disease can be determined.
- More than one outcome can be considered
- This design allows the risk of disease to be measured directly
- It is possible, given sufficient resources, to measure information about exposure to risk factors in detail and also to examine exposure to a range of risk factors
- There is likely to be less chance of recall and selection bias than in case-control studies
- Exposure is measured prior to the outcome and so helps avoid bias.

Disadvantages of cohort studies

- Because the participants have to be followed up for a long period of time, cohort studies are expensive to conduct
- If the disease or condition is rare, it is necessary to follow up with a large number of individuals (hence, case-control studies are generally better for investigating rare conditions)
- Loss of participants over time can introduce bias. This is particularly a problem if the loss is linked to a risk factor
- It is important to maintain consistency of measuring either exposure to the risk factor or the disease of interest for the duration of the study (which may, in some cases, be years)

Box 14.1 Example of a cohort study

Differential unmet needs and experience of restorative dental care in trajectories of dental caries experience: a birth cohort study.

Ruiz et al. (2023) Caries Research. 1, 2023, May 22. https://doi.org/10.1159/000530378.

Dental caries is a chronic and cumulative disease, but little has been reported on the continuity of the disease and its treatment throughout life. Group-based multi-trajectory modelling was used to identify developmental trajectories of untreated carious tooth surfaces (DS), restored tooth surfaces (FS), and teeth extracted due to caries (MT) from ages 9–45 years in a New Zealand longitudinal birth cohort, the Dunedin Multidisciplinary Health and Development Study ($n = 975$). Associations between early life risk factors and trajectory group membership were examined by specifying the probability of group membership according to a multinomial logit model. Six trajectory groups were identified and labelled: 'low caries rate'; 'moderate caries rate, maintained'; 'moderate caries rate, unmaintained'; 'high caries rate, restored'; 'high caries rate, tooth loss'; and 'high caries rate, untreated caries'. The two moderate-caries-rate groups differed in a count of FS. The three high-caries-rate groups differed in the relative proportion of accumulated DS, FS, and MT. Early childhood risk factors associated with less favourable trajectories included higher dmfs scores at age five, lack of exposure to community water fluoridation during the first five years of life, lower childhood IQ, and low childhood socioeconomic status. Parent self-ratings of their own or their child's oral health as 'poor' were associated with less favourable caries experience trajectories. Children with clinical signs of dental caries and a parent rating of the child's oral health as poor were more likely to follow a less favourable caries trajectory. Higher deciduous dentition caries experience at age five years was associated with less favourable caries trajectories, as were children whose parents gave 'poor' ratings of their own or their child's oral health. These findings highlight the considerable intergenerational continuity in dental caries risk and experience from early childhood to midlife. Subjective measures of child oral health are informative and might aid as predictors of adult caries experience in cases where childhood dental clinical data were unavailable.

Source: *Ruiz et al. (2023) Reproduced with permission from Karger.*

- Disease outcome or risk factors may themselves change over time.

An example of a cohort study is shown in Box 14.1. This study involved a cohort of just over 1000 individuals born in Dunedin, New Zealand, in 1972/1973 who have been followed since birth. This report examines the patterns of dental caries development from age 9 to age 45 years in 975 individuals. Using this study design, it is possible to see how factors present at the beginning of the observation period impact how dental caries rates and patterns developed over the subsequent 36 years.

Randomised controlled trials

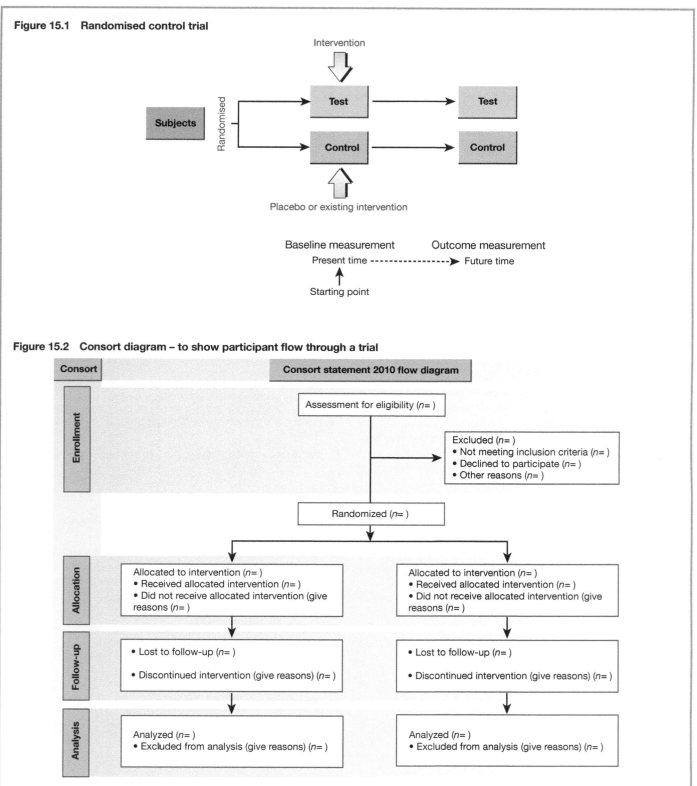

Figure 15.1   Randomised control trial

Figure 15.2   Consort diagram – to show participant flow through a trial

Dental Public Health at a Glance, Second Edition. Ivor G. Chestnutt.
© 2024 John Wiley & Sons Ltd. Published 2024 by John Wiley & Sons Ltd.

A randomised controlled trial (RCT) is an **interventional study** and is **prospective** in nature (Figure 15.1). Study participants are identified according to predefined inclusion criteria. The participants are then randomly assigned to either a **test** or **control group**. The test group then receives the intervention under test, while the control group receives no intervention, a **placebo** intervention or an existing treatment. The participants are followed for a period of time, and the **outcome** is measured at the end. The change from baseline in both test and control groups is measured. The test and control groups are then compared to determine whether there is any **difference in outcome** in the test and control groups. In this way, a conclusion can be reached on whether the intervention or treatment applied to the test group had a more desirable outcome than the intervention received by the control group.

Analysis of a randomised controlled trial

The type of analysis undertaken in a randomised controlled trial will depend on the nature of the outcome measure used. The general principle is the application of a statistical test to determine whether the difference in outcome observed between the test and control group at the end of the study is likely to have occurred by chance or is likely to be a true difference.

It is then necessary to determine whether the difference is of **clinical significance**. It is possible for the difference to be statistically significant – that is, for it to be true and not simply have occurred by chance. However, it is possible that the difference is small and not likely to be of greater clinical benefit over the intervention received by the control group.

Advantages of randomised controlled trials

• Are considered the 'gold standard' of study design, largely because of the degree to which they can control for bias and confounding factors
• Allow randomisation and can therefore minimise the effect of confounding
• Can be 'blind' and therefore minimise the effect of bias
• Are often multicentre – that is, participants are recruited from more than one site
• Participants in RCTs get excellent care (even if in the control group).

Disadvantages of randomised controlled trials

• Expensive to conduct
• Require specialist skills to organise and conduct
• Recruitment of sufficient numbers of study participants in a defined period of time can be a challenge
• Participants can be lost to follow-up
• RCTs can only be used to examine interventions with a positive outcome for the participants.

It is unethical to use an RCT design to examine the aetiology of disease. So, for example, while it is appropriate to test the anti-caries effect of fluoride-containing toothpaste in an RCT, it would be unethical to demonstrate the cariogenic effect of sugar using an RCT design.

Issues relating to randomised controlled trials

Randomisation

The term 'random' in RCT relates to the manner in which participants are allocated to either the test or control group. Each participant should have an equal chance of being allocated or **randomised** to the test or control group.

Usually, participants are randomised on an individual basis. However, sometimes participants are randomised in groups or 'clusters', for example, schools or classrooms within a school. **Cluster randomised controlled trials** will require more participants, and the clustering effect needs to be accounted for in the analysis of the trial outcome.

Stratification

While individuals are allocated to a trial arm at random, it is important that before the trial begins, the test and control groups are as alike as possible. For example, in a clinical trial of fluoride-containing toothpaste, the test and control groups should not differ significantly in terms of caries prevalence, number of males and females or the age of participants. This is achieved by a process called **stratification**. In critically appraising a clinical trial, it is important to look for a table that, at **baseline,** compares important possible confounding factors between test and control groups.

Blinding

Blinding (or allocation concealment) is the process whereby the study group to which a participant is allocated is hidden from the participant, the experimenter conducting the outcome measurement or both. When only the participant is unaware of the intervention they are receiving, this is known as '**single blind**'. When both participant and experimenter are unaware, this is known as '**double blind**'. In a '**triple-blind**' study, the statistician conducting the analysis is also unaware of which of the groups is receiving the test intervention and which is receiving the control intervention.

Trial arm

The term 'arm' describes a group receiving the same intervention. In a classical clinical trial, there are two arms: the test group and the control group (Figure 15.1). However, some trials can have more than two arms – as many as six in some studies, although these require large numbers of participants.

Training and calibration

It is important that the experimenters measure the study outcome in a reproducible and consistent manner. To achieve this, the clinicians recording the study outcome undergo training in the use of the instrument or index (Chapter 4) employed to measure the outcome. To ensure that they are scoring the outcome in a similar fashion, a **calibration exercise** is carried out where the examiners all measure the same patient or photograph of an outcome measure. The level of agreement among the examiners can be determined statistically and is reported as a Kappa score. A score of 1 indicates perfect agreement (this seldom occurs), and a score of 0 represents no agreement. Calibration of examiners is particularly important when study participants are recruited at multiple sites. For example, the BRIGHT clinical trial (Marshman et al. 2019) examined the use of SMS messages to encourage toothbrushing in adolescents recruited across Britain. All of the examiners must assess the outcomes in a consistent fashion.

The CONSORT standard for reporting RCTs is outlined in Figure 15.2. The CONSORT-Outcomes 2022 extension of the CONSORT 2010 statement provides 17 outcome-specific items that should be addressed in all published clinical trial reports to increase trial utility, replicability and transparency and may minimise the risk of selective nonreporting of trial results.

16 Randomised controlled trials II: Split mouth and cross-over studies

Figure 16.1 Diagrammatic representation of a split-mouth randomised controlled trial. Restorative material A placed on right hand side in 50% of study participants and on left hand side in 50% (vice-versa with material B). Both materials are therefore tested in the same oral environment

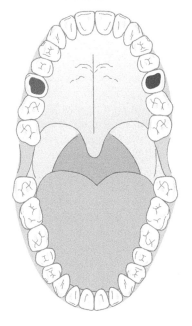 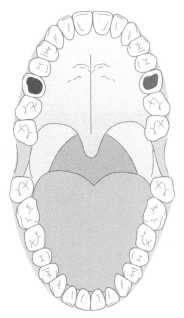

Figure 16.2 Diagrammatic representation of a cross-over study

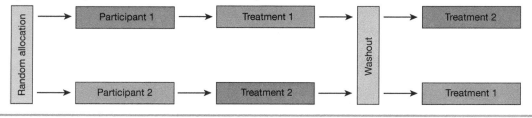

Dental Public Health at a Glance, Second Edition. Ivor G. Chestnutt.
© 2024 John Wiley & Sons Ltd. Published 2024 by John Wiley & Sons Ltd.

In addition to the conventional parallel, two-arm randomised controlled trial (Chapter 15, Figure 15.1), there are two other forms of interventional study design that are encountered in dental research. These are both forms of controlled clinical trials in which the participants act as both test and control: a split-mouth trial and a cross-over trial.

Split mouth clinical trial

In a study of this design, a participant receives two interventions simultaneously, the test on one side of the mouth and the control on the contralateral (same arch, opposite side) or ipsilateral (opposite arch, same side) side (Figure 16.1). The side that receives the test treatment is decided randomly, but overall, 50% of participants will have the test intervention on the right side and 50% on the left. This minimises any effect of bias due to the treatment being on the left- or right-hand side. Occasionally, the control site may be ipsilateral (i.e. test sites are in the mandible and maxilla on the same side of the mouth). Some studies have tested four interventions, one in each quadrant of the mouth. Split mouth studies are most useful for investigating restorative dental materials. It is important that 'cross-over' effects are considered before utilising a split-mouth design. For example, it would not be appropriate to test a fluoride-releasing glass-ionomer restorative material in a split-mouth study. Fluoride leach may affect the control site on the contra- or ipsilateral side.

Advantages of a split-mouth trial

• Test and control interventions tested in the same intraoral environment, thereby helping to control confounding factors
• Fewer participants are needed.

Disadvantages of a split-mouth trial

• Statistical analysis needs to account for the fact that the sites are clustered/nested within one individual and are therefore not independent, and paired tests should be used
• Need to recruit participants who require the intervention in two contra- (or ipsilateral) sites.

An example of a split-mouth study can be found in Box 16.1.

Cross-over trial

In a study of this design, the participant receives both test and control treatment, but in series; that is, one after the other. An

---

Box 16.1 Example of a split-mouth study

Time to complain about pain. Children's self-reported procedural pain in a randomised control trial of Hall and conventional stainless steel crown techniques.
Boyd, D.H. et al. (2023) International Journal Paediatric Dentistry 33:382–393.
Aim: To investigate procedural pain scores for two treatments for carious primary molars in New Zealand primary care.
Design: This study was a split-mouth randomised control trial with secondary outcome analysis. Children (4–8 years) with proximal carious lesions on matched primary molars had one tooth treated with the Hall technique (HT) and one treated with a conventional stainless steel crown (CT); treatment type and order of treatment were randomly allocated. The Wong–Baker self-report pain scale measured pre-treatment dental pain, procedural pain at each treatment and post-operative pain.
Results: Data were analysed for 103 children: 49 children had the HT first, and 54 children had the CT first. Procedural pain scores did not differ by treatment type, with 71.8% and 76.7% of children reporting low pain for the HT and the CT, respectively.

Box 16.2 Example of a cross-over study

Effect of thickness and occlusal accommodation on the degree of satisfaction with mouthguard use among water polo players: A randomised crossover trial.
Flores-Figueiras C. et al. (2020) Dental Traumatology. 36: 670–679.
Aim: To assess the effect of using a thicker custom-made mouthguard with occlusal accommodation on the degree of satisfaction among water polo players.
Material and Methods: Twenty-five elite water polo players participated in this randomised crossover trial. For each participant, two customised mouthguards were fabricated using 4-mm ethyl vinyl acetate foil: Type A included no occlusal accommodation and Type B included a 2-mm occlusal accommodation. Players wore each mouthguard during training sessions and competitions for two weeks in one of two randomised sequences. After each match or training session, players were asked to evaluate the mouthguards.
Results: The mouthguard with occlusal accommodation was reported to interfere more with speech and swallowing and with aesthetics, breathing, and athletic performance compared with the conventional mouthguard. Although occlusal accommodation was associated with a higher perceived degree of protection, players were still more satisfied with the conventional mouthguard.

---

example would be a study on the anti-calculus properties of toothpaste (Figure 16.2). Following a scale and polish, the study participant uses the test toothpaste for a period (in this example, about three months) and the amount of new calculus that has developed is measured. The participant then uses a standard toothpaste for a period (in this example, one month) to allow any 'hangover' effects of the test product to dissipate. Following a further scale and polish, the participant then used the control toothpaste for a similar period to that for which they used the test treatment. The amount of new calculus that has been developed is measured and compared with the test product. One-half of the study participants will receive the test toothpaste first, while the other half will have the control product first to minimise any order effects.

Advantages of a cross-over trial

• Test and control interventions are tested in the same participants, so fewer participants are required
• Patients act as their own control, so confounding factors are minimised.

Disadvantages of a cross-over trial

• Can only be used to test outcomes that are recurrent and reversible, e.g. accumulation of dental plaque and calculus
• Results are nested within participants, so more complex statistical analysis is required
• Because treatments are tested in series (i.e. one after the other), the study lasts longer than a parallel study design.

An example of a cross-over study can be found in Box 16.2.
Box 16.3 describes an analysis of randomised controlled trials.

Box 16.3 Analysis of randomised controlled trials

Per protocol analysis – At the conclusion of an RCT, only those participants who adhered to the published protocol are included in the analysis.
Intention to treat analysis – At the conclusion of an RCT, the outcome data for all participants (when available) is analysed according to the group to which they were allocated, irrespective of whether or not they adhered strictly to the trial protocol. This is the preferred form of analysis as it is less likely to introduce bias and also more likely to be reflective of 'real world' results. The main difficulty is having available outcome data for participants who fail to complete the trial.

Systematic reviews and meta-analysis

Figure 17.1 Forest plot – used to present the outcome of meta-analysis

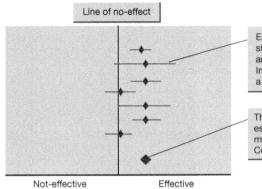

Line of no-effect

Studies with mean to the left of no-effect line indicate intervention not effective

In this example seven studies contributed to the meta-analysis. five suggested a positive effect, two studies suggested no effect. Overall the meta-analysis suggests a definite positive effect

Each horizontal line represents a single study, the diamond is the mean odds ratio and the line represents the 95% Confidence Interval. Wide confidence intervals suggest a study with small number of participants

This large diamond represents the overall estimate effect. The centre of the diamond is mean effect, the width is the overall 95% Confidence Interval

Not-effective   Effective

Figure 17.2 PRISMA flow diagram

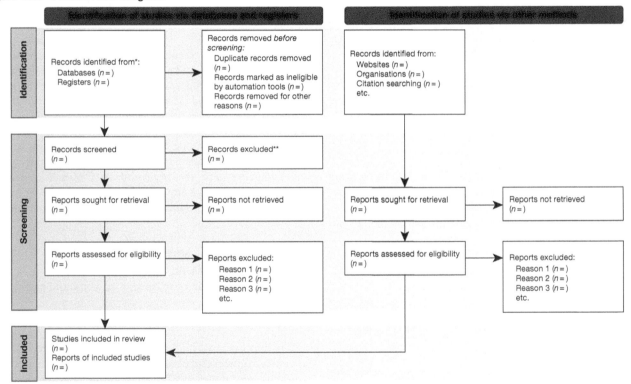

Identification of studies via databases and registers

Identification

Records identified from*:
Databases (*n* =)
Registers (*n* =)

Records removed *before screening:*
Duplicate records removed (*n* =)
Records marked as ineligible by automation tools (*n* =)
Records removed for other reasons (*n* =)

Identification of studies via other methods

Records identified from:
Websites (*n* =)
Organisations (*n* =)
Citation searching (*n* =)
etc.

Screening

Records screened (*n* =)

Records excluded** (*n* =)

Reports sought for retrieval (*n* =)

Reports not retrieved (*n* =)

Reports assessed for eligibility (*n* =)

Reports excluded:
Reason 1 (*n* =)
Reason 2 (*n* =)
Reason 3 (*n* =)
etc.

Reports sought for retrieval (*n* =)

Reports not retrieved (*n* =)

Reports assessed for eligibility (*n* =)

Reports excluded:
Reason 1 (*n* =)
Reason 2 (*n* =)
Reason 3 (*n* =)
etc.

Included

Studies included in review (*n* =)
Reports of included studies (*n* =)

Figure 17.3 Funnel plot

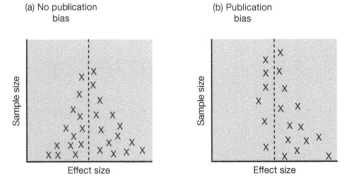

(a) No publication bias

(b) Publication bias

Sample size

Effect size

Sample size

Effect size

Publication bias (Figure 17.3) – occurs when only a part of the existing data are available.
Publication can occur because journals are more likely to publish positive results and researchers may not seek publication of negative results.
The presence of publication bias can be detected using a funnel plot.
A funnel plot which is symmetrical about the mean and looks like an upside down funnel suggests no publication bias (a).
When the bottom left portion of the plot is missing– publication bias should be suspected (b).
The detection of publication bias is useful in interpreting the evidence but difficult to correct for.

Dental Public Health at a Glance, Second Edition. Ivor G. Chestnutt.
© 2024 John Wiley & Sons Ltd. Published 2024 by John Wiley & Sons Ltd.

Systematic review

A systematic review is a form of secondary research in which existing information is searched for in a highly organised fashion according to a predefined protocol. Efforts are made to identify not only information published in standard academic journals, but also that from the 'grey literature', not controlled by commercial publishers. Data are extracted from individual studies. Provided that a common outcome measure has been used and that there are sufficient studies, data can be combined statistically (meta-analysis) to give an overall effect. The typical steps in conducting a systematic review are shown in Table 17.1.

Advantages of systematic reviews

• Provide an overall summary of the effectiveness of an intervention or contribution of a risk factor to a disease/condition
• Include the 'grey literature', unpublished studies
• Include studies published in languages other than English
• Overcome bias inherent in traditional narrative reviews, where the search strategy, inclusion and exclusion criteria and method for reaching a conclusion are not transparent
• Development and use have been greatly encouraged by the Cochrane Collaboration (Chapter 18).

Limitations of systematic reviews

• Are reliant on a sufficient number of studies having been conducted with a similar outcome measure
• The proper conduct of a systematic review requires researchers with a range of skills, e.g. literature search skills, as well as statisticians, research methodologists and clinicians.

Table 17.1 Steps in conducting a systematic review

Stage	Process
Identify the topic for review and agree a clearly defined research question(s)	It is important to identify a clearly defined question of clinical relevance, e.g. is fluoride varnish effective in preventing dental caries? Check whether a systematic review on this topic has already been carried out. If so, is it up to date?
Draft the protocol for the review	This should be very clear on how the review will be conducted and should clearly describe the: • research question • search strategy • inclusion and exclusion criteria for studies • protocol for data extraction • approach to the statistical analysis of the data.
The search strategy	This is likely to be in several parts: • **Formal review** of the published literature. Help should be sought from an experienced librarian/information technologist to formulate the search strategy. This will need to define the bibliographic databases to be searched, e.g. Medline, EMBASE and CINAHL, and will vary according to the research question. The keywords and combination of keywords for the search will need to be agreed. The publication time frame for included studies will need to be defined, as will the languages of the studies to be included – either restricted to English or more useful to include all languages. • **Hand search:** This involves screening the index pages of relevant journals to identify relevant studies that might not have been identified by the formal electronic search. Although called a hand search, this is conducted by looking at the index pages of the online version of relevant journals. • **Reference list/bibliography search:** The reference lists of relevant studies identified earlier are read to identify any studies not picked up in the original review. This is called **citation changing**. • **Grey literature:** This describes data that has not been formally published and may include data held by product manufacturers, data on websites, or data held by academics that has not been formally published. • **Specific call for information:** Occasionally, researchers conducting a systematic review will set up a website to which data may be submitted.
Identification of relevant studies	Following the search, the titles and abstracts of studies selected are screened to identify possible relevant studies – many of the studies identified by the searches will not meet the inclusion criteria. For example, in a systematic review of the effects of fluoride varnish, studies that were not in the form of a randomised controlled trial would be excluded.
Data extraction	Data from the studies identified as relevant are extracted and entered into a specifically designed database. So, in the case of the systematic review on the clinical effectiveness of fluoride varnish, the magnitude of the caries increment in test and control groups would be noted, together with other relevant information, such as whether this was in primary or permanent teeth, the duration of the study, the frequency of the varnish application, the number of participants in the study.
Data analysis – meta-analysis	Provided that there are sufficient studies using the same outcome measure, the outcome measure can be combined via an advanced statistical technique called a **meta-analysis**. This gives an overall idea of the effectiveness of the intervention being reviewed, and is reported using a **forest plot** (Figure 17.1). A major consideration is the heterogeneity of the studies to be included in the meta-analysis. Heterogeneity exists where the variation in the estimates of the treatment effects reported by individual studies to be included in the systematic review is greater than would have been expected by chance. When a meta-analysis is not possible, a narrative review may be presented. Here, the results are described in words, without a formal statistical estimate of the combined effects.
Reporting	Guidance on how to report a systematic review is provided by the PRISMA statement (Figure 17.2). This comprises a 27-statement checklist and a 4-phase flow diagram (www.prisma-statement.org/). **PRISMA** stands for **Preferred Reporting Items for Systematic Reviews and Meta-Analyses**.

18 Evidence-based dentistry and clinical guidelines

Figure 18.1   The WHO health gain rhomboid

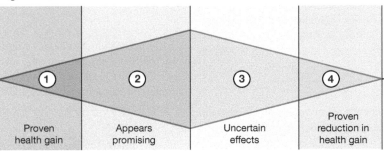

| 1 | 2 | 3 | 4 |

| Proven health gain | Appears promising | Uncertain effects | Proven reduction in health gain |

Figure 18.2   The components of evidence-based practice

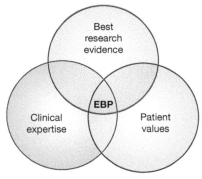

Evidence-based practice

In 1972, Professor Archie Cochrane, who is now regarded as the 'father' of the evidence-based healthcare movement, published a document called 'Effectiveness and efficiency – random reflections on health services'. The basic tenet of Cochrane's observations was that in providing healthcare, efforts should be made to encourage the use of practices and procedures shown by scientific studies to provide a positive health gain. At the same time, interventions that are of no benefit or are harmful should not be used.

In 1996, Sackett and colleagues defined evidence-based practice as:

The conscientious, explicit and judicious use of current best evidence in making decisions about the care of individual patients. The practice of evidence-based medicine means integrating individual clinical expertise with the best available external clinical evidence from systematic research.

Evidence-based dentistry

By inference, evidence-based dentistry can be defined as follows:

Evidence-based dentistry is the practice of dentistry that integrates the best available evidence with clinical experience and patient preference in making clinical decisions.

The health gain rhomboid (Figure 18.1) categorises treatments and procedures into one of four categories. The argument is that many treatments currently provided fall into categories 2 and 3, where their benefits are either promising or uncertain – but they have not been proven to be the most effective and efficient way to provide care. The aim of evidence-based practice is to deliver more and more treatments that are categorised in category 1; that is, they have been shown by scientific studies to result in positive health gain. Procedures that result in harm to patients (category 4) should not be provided. While this seems obvious, there are numerous examples in the healthcare literature of procedures that continued to be provided even after they had been proven to be ineffective or, even worse to be harmful.

In its guidance to members of the dental team, the General Dental Council requires the provision of quality care based on up-to-date evidence.

The Cochrane Collaboration

The Cochrane Collaboration (named in honour of Archie Cochrane) is an independent global network of researchers, clinicians, patients and individuals interested in healthcare whose mission is to promote evidence-informed health decision-making by producing high-quality, relevant, accessible, systematic reviews and other synthesised research evidence.

Dental Public Health at a Glance, Second Edition. Ivor G. Chestnutt.
© 2024 John Wiley & Sons Ltd. Published 2024 by John Wiley & Sons Ltd.

The most tangible aspect of the Cochrane Collaboration is the Cochrane Library (www.cochranelibrary.com). This contains over 200 systematic reviews of relevance to dental and oral health.

Clinical guidelines

Given the vast number of research studies published in any week, month or year, it is impossible for a busy clinician to keep up to date by reading and making sense of the original research articles. This is complicated by the fact that the articles will often have conflicting or equivocal results. Clinical guidelines have been developed to help overcome this problem.

Clinical guidelines attempt to synthesise the current evidence base in a format that can be read by healthcare providers. Used in conjunction with the clinician's personal experience and expertise and the patient's preferences, the hope is that the guidelines will inform evidence-based decisions and choices of treatment (Figure 18.2).

Guideline producers

National Institute for Health and Care Excellence (NICE)

The National Institute for Health and Care Excellence (NICE) (www.nice.org.uk) is a non-departmental public body, which, while accountable to the Department of Health in England, is independent of government. NICE aims are to improve outcomes for people using the NHS and other public health and social care services. The functions of NICE include:

• producing evidence-based guidance and advice for health, public health and social care practitioners
• developing quality standards and performance metrics for those providing and commissioning health, public health and social care services
• providing a range of informational services for commissioners, practitioners and managers across the spectrum of health and social care.

NICE has produced guidelines of relevance to both clinical and dental public health practice (Table 18.1).

Scottish Dental Clinical Effectiveness Programme (SDCEP)

The Scottish Dental Clinical Effectiveness Programme part of NHS Scotland produces guidelines relevant to dentistry (Table 18.1).

Specialist societies

A number of specialist dental societies have produced guidelines of relevance to clinical practice with their area of interest (Table 18.1).

Certainty of the evidence

Guidelines often grade the level of evidence. This indicates where on the hierarchy of evidence (Table 11.1) the source of the guidance originates. For example, is it high-level evidence derived from a systematic review and meta-analysis, or is it merely an expert opinion adopted without robust evidence from formal research studies.

A number of systems have been proposed to classify the certainty of evidence. One of the most commonly used is the **GRADE (Grading of Recommendations, Assessment, Development and Evaluation)** system of rating the quality of evidence and grading strength of recommendations in systematic reviews, health technology assessments (HTAs), and clinical practice guidelines addressing alternative management options (Siemieniuk and Guyatt 2023) (Table 18.2). After the evidence is collected and summarised, GRADE provides explicit criteria for rating the quality of evidence that include study design, risk of bias, imprecision, inconsistency, indirectness, and magnitude of effect (Table 18.3).

Recommendations are characterised as strong or weak (alternative terms conditional or discretionary) according to the quality of the supporting evidence and the balance between desirable and undesirable consequences of the alternative management options. Evidence derived from randomised controlled trials is generally regarded as of the greatest quality. However, in some instances (e.g. in chronic diseases with long-term outcomes such as atherosclerosis, it is accepted that observational studies are acceptable as forms of evidence). GRADE is subjective and arrived at by consensus of the individuals making the recommendations.

Table 18.1 Examples of clinical guidelines of relevance to dentistry

Guideline producer	Guideline title
British Orthodontic Society	A Guideline for the Extraction of First Permanent Molars in Children
British Society of Periodontology	Guidelines for Periodontal Screening and Management of Children and Adolescents under 18 Years of Age
National Institute for Health and Care Excellence (NICE)	Dental Checks: Intervals Between Oral Health Reviews
National Institute for Health and Care Excellence (NICE)	Guidance on the Extraction of Wisdom Teeth
National Institute for Health and Care Excellence (NICE)	Oral Health: Local Authorities and Partners
National Institute for Health and Care Excellence (NICE)	Oral Health for Adults in Care Homes
National Institute for Health and Care Excellence (NICE)	Oral Health Promotion: General Dental Practice
Scottish Dental Clinical Effectiveness Programme	Dental Caries in Children

Table 18.2 GRADE certainty ratings

Certainty	What it means
Very low	The true effect is probably markedly different from the estimated effect
Low	The true effect might be markedly different from the estimated effect
Moderate	The authors believe that the true effect is probably close to the estimated effect
High	The authors have a lot of confidence that the true effect is similar to the estimated effect

Source: *Siemieniuk and Guyatt (2023)/BMJ Publishing Group Limited. https://bestpractice.bmj.com/info/toolkit/learn-ebm/what-is-grade/ (with permission).*

Table 18.3 Reasons certainty in rating evidence can be moved up or down when using the GRADE assessment system

Certainty can be rated down for:	Certainty can be rated up for:
• Risk of bias	• The large magnitude of the effect
• Imprecision	• Dose-response gradient
• Inconsistency	• All residual confounding would decrease the magnitude of the effect (in situations with an effect).
• Indirectness	
• Publication bias	

Source: *Siemieniuk and Guyatt (2023)/BMJ Publishing Group Limited. https://bestpractice.bmj.com/info/toolkit/learn-ebm/what-is-grade/ (with permission).*

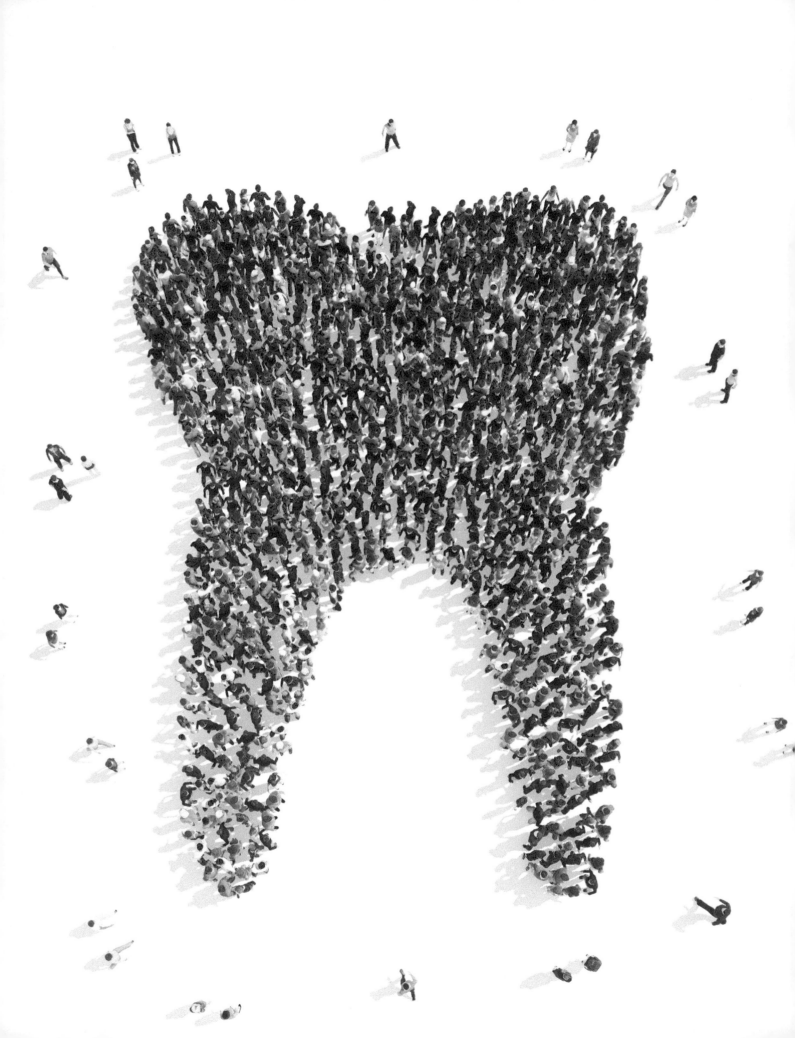

Oral health promotion

Part 4

Chapters

19 Inequalities in oral health

Figure 19.1   dmft at age five years by deprivation quintile (Wales 2015–2016)

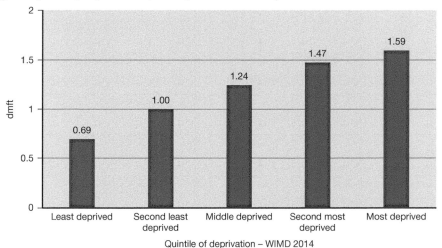

WIMD = Wales Index of Multiple Deprivation

Figure 19.2   The distribution of dental caries in five-year-old children (Wales 2015–2016)

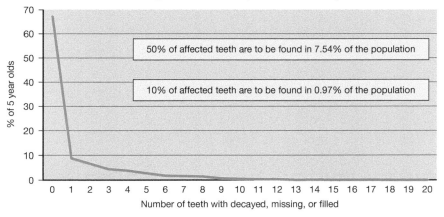

50% of affected teeth are to be found in 7.54% of the population

10% of affected teeth are to be found in 0.97% of the population

Figure 19.3   Diagrammatic representation of desirable and undesirable changes in the prevalence of the disease by deprivation category following the implementation of an oral health improvement programme

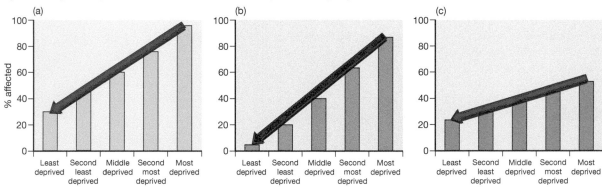

Diagrammatic representation of how oral health improvement programmes may affect health inequalities.

(a) Situation where disease prevalence is directly proportional to deprivation status (purple line)

(b) Represents the inequality gradient where implementation of an oral health improvement programme has disproportionately advantaged the least deprived - thereby widening the gap between least and most deprived - an undesirable consequence (red line)

(c) Represents the situation where an oral health improvement programme has favoured the most deprived quintiles thereby reducing oral health inequalities - a desired consequence (green line)

The determinants of health were, described in Chapter 2, and the significant gains in oral health observed in the United Kingdom in children and adults over the past four decades were discussed in Chapter 9. However, the improvements in oral health have not been equally distributed across the population. In common with most lifestyle-influenced diseases, oral diseases are heavily influenced by social and economic status.

Measuring social and economic status

Social class

The concept of classifying the population based on social and economic status dates back to the 1850s. By the early twentieth century, a measure of social class based on the occupation of the head of the household had been devised by the Registrar General's Office in the United Kingdom. This worked well for the first eight decades of the twentieth century. However, as working patterns and family structures changed, the occupational status of one individual in a household increasingly failed to reflect the growing number of families where two adults worked or where there was just one adult.

Area-based measures of deprivation

The limitations of social class as a measure of deprivation have led to the development of area-based measures. These relate not to an individual family but to the neighbourhood where the family lives – an area that includes about 1500 people. This is called a Lower Layer Super Output Area (LLSOA). There are 32844 LLSOAs in England and 1909 in Wales. For each LLSOA, seven domains are measured (Table 19.1). These can be employed either separately or in combination to give a measure of relative deprivation (i.e. how deprived one locality is in relation to another). Using a patient's postcode, it is possible to determine the relative deprivation of where they live.

There are Indices of Multiple Deprivation for England, Scotland and Wales. To examine how disease prevalence relates to deprivation, it is possible to segment (divide up) the population into equal fifths (quintiles), sevenths (septiles) or tenths (deciles). For example, Figure 19.1 shows how dental caries varies according to the quintile of deprivation in Welsh five-year-olds.

Reports on deprivation and health

There have been several prominent reports on the relationship between deprivation and health. *Fair Society, Healthy Lives* (the Marmot Report), published in 2010, set a number of indicators of the social determinants of health, health outcomes and social inequality and recommended actions to address health inequalities (Table 19.2). A 2020 review of progress in addressing health inequalities concluded that much remained to be done and in fact some aspects of health inequalities had worsened in the 2010s (Table 19.3).

Inequalities in oral health

Children

Figure 5.5 demonstrates how the distribution of dental caries in populations has changed from being normally distributed to a skewed distribution where the disease is concentrated in fewer

Table 19.1 The domains that contribute to the Index of Multiple Deprivation

- Income
- Employment
- Health
- Education, skills and training
- Barriers to housing and services.

Table 19.2 Marmot indicators 2014 – actions to address health inequalities based on the Marmot Review (2010)

- Give every child the best start in life
- Enable all children, young people and adults to maximise their capabilities and have control over their lives
- Create fair employment and good work for all
- Ensure a healthy standard of living for all
- Create and develop healthy and sustainable places and communities
- Strengthen the role and impact of ill-health prevention.

Table 19.3 Health equity in England: The Marmot Review 10 years on (2020)

A follow-up review of the 2010 report in 2020 concluded that:
- Since 2010, life expectancy in England has stalled for the first time since 1900
- The amount of time people spend in poor health has increased across England since 2010
- People in deprived communities not only die sooner, but spend a greater proportion of their shorter lives in poor health than those from less deprived communities
- There are marked regional differences in life expectancy, particularly among people living in more deprived areas.

individuals from more deprived backgrounds. The distribution of dental caries in Welsh five-year-olds is illustrated in Figure 19.2. This demonstrates that 67% are caries-free and that the disease is confined to 33% of the population. This distribution shows the 'high-risk' tail to the distribution, with 10% of carious teeth concentrated in just 1% of the population.

Adults

The 2009 Adult Dental Health Survey concluded that oral health inequalities manifest in different ways in different age groups, representing age and cohort effects. So, while there were no differences in the number of missing teeth by social class in younger adults, in older adults, the least deprived had 4.5 fewer teeth missing than the most deprived.

In oral disease, where the risk factors are heavily linked to social class, such as oral cancer, differences in disease prevalence across social divides are large. Not only is oral cancer more common in those from deprived backgrounds, but adults from lower social classes are more likely to present to a doctor or dentist when the cancer is at a more advanced stage and, therefore, with a poorer prognosis (Chapter 7).

Quantifying health inequalities

Figure 19.3 demonstrates the gradient in oral health across quintiles of deprivation (i.e. the population divided into equal fifths). A measure called the Slope Index of Inequality can be used to quantify the degree of difference across social classes. It represents the linear regression coefficient of the relation between the level of disease in each socio-economic category and the hierarchical ranking of each socio-economic category on the social scale (Figure 19.3a).

Addressing oral health inequalities

The aim of health improvement programmes should be to address inequalities in oral health. This requires careful consideration. The provision of a programme that is only taken up by those at the upper end and middle of the social spectrum has the potential to widen oral health inequalities (Figure 19.3b). Ideally, health improvement programmes should have a maximal effect on the most deprived, thereby flattening the inequality slope (Figure 19.3c). Strategic approaches to improving oral health are discussed further in Chapter 24.

20 Oral health education, oral health promotion and oral health improvement

Figure 20.1 Health promotion – a combination of health education, prevention and health protection

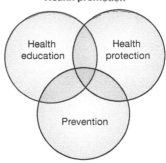

Health promotion

Health education

Health protection

Prevention

Figure 20.2 The concept of upstream and downstream approaches to oral health improvement

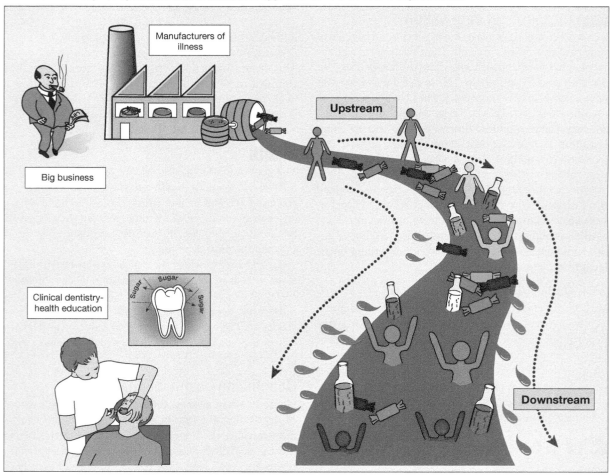

Preventing disease and improving health is one of the three key objectives of public health. The other two are improving services and health protection (preventing infectious diseases and environmental hazards).

Health improvement requires a key understanding of the determinants of health (Chapter 2). Securing health involves action at different levels – *the individual, professional health and care services,* and *society.* The balance between these aspects and where responsibility for preventing disease and securing health lies are frequently debated. As an example, in the prevention of dental caries, should the responsibility lie with individuals who, by reducing the frequency of sugar consumption and brushing their teeth with fluoride toothpaste, markedly reduce their caries risk, or should individuals be helped by the government imposing a tax on sugared drinks and implementing water fluoridation?

Dental Public Health at a Glance, Second Edition. Ivor G. Chestnutt.
© 2024 John Wiley & Sons Ltd. Published 2024 by John Wiley & Sons Ltd.

Health promotion is an all-encompassing concept that, in addition to health education, includes health protection and prevention (Figure 20.1).

Health education provides information to individuals and populations on how to prevent disease and improve health.

Health protection comprises laws, regulations, policies and voluntary codes of practice aimed at preventing disease and enhancing health, for instance, seat-belt laws or no-smoking policies.

Prevention includes patient-based interventions such as fissure sealants or application of fluoride varnish.

Approaches to health improvement

Oral health education

There are six key messages in securing oral health and preventing dental disease (Table 20.1). It is important that individuals understand and act on these messages. Dental professionals have an important role to play in delivering these messages on a one-to-one basis at the chairside. This is one of the few opportunities when individuals can have the messages tailored to their own particular needs and circumstances.

Limitations of oral health education

While oral health education is important on a one-to-one basis, it has a number of limitations:

• **Knowledge, attitudes and behaviour:** Changes in knowledge do not necessarily lead to changes in behaviour. Education may enhance knowledge and alter an individual's attitude and desire to live more healthily. However, this does not mean that they will necessarily change their behaviour. So, an individual may know that smoking is detrimental to their periodontal health and may want to stop smoking, but the effort involved, plus the addiction to nicotine, may prevent them from changing their behaviour and stopping smoking.

• **Short-term improvements:** even if an individual manages to change their behaviour, this is often short-lived – New Year's resolutions are a typical example of how well-intentioned actions to engage in health behaviours may not last more than a few days or weeks.

• **Personal circumstances may preclude action:** eating a diet rich in fruit and vegetables – the 5-a-day message – may be difficult for a family from a disadvantaged background where cost, access and cooking skills may well inhibit them from taking up this recommendation.

• **Medical model outdated:** often health promotion messages promote health only in terms of the absence of disease, and the wider dimensions of health are ignored.

• **Negative – disease-focused, victim blaming:** many health education messages are negative, focusing on what people should not do rather than on what they should.

• **Directive:** many health education messages are dictatorial and fail to recognise people's individual life circumstances.

Table 20.1 The key messages for oral health education

• **Diet:** reduce both the amount and frequency of intake of sugar-containing food and drink – 'Eat less sugar and eat sugar less often'
• **Toothbrushing:** clean your teeth thoroughly twice every day with a fluoride toothpaste
• **Dental attendance:** have a regular oral examination at a time interval recommended by your dentist, based on your risk of oral disease
• **Mouthguards:** Always wear a custom-made mouthguard when participating in contact sports
• **Tobacco:** do not smoke tobacco or use tobacco in any other form
• **Alcohol:** consume alcohol in moderation and keep to the recommended weekly limits. Have alcohol-free days each week and do not binge drink

• **Potential to widen inequalities in health:** inappropriately applied health education that is only acted on by the least deprived has the potential to widen oral health inequalities (Figure 19.3).
• **Conflicting messages:** contradictory messages, often promoted by the media who like controversial stories, can confuse the public and undo years of good work by disrupting public understanding of the evidence.
• **Limited evidence of benefit in group settings:** although talks to parents and children in schools have traditionally been undertaken by dental educators. However, in the absence of an intervention involving the provision of fluoride there is little evidence that classroom health education is effective. A recent trial involving SMS text messages to promote toothbrushing failed to demonstrate a clinical benefit in reducing dental caries.

The Ottawa Charter

Health education was the traditional approach to improving health. It has an important role on a one-to-one basis but has limited potential on a population basis. Probably the most influential development in the field of health improvement was the production of the Ottawa Charter in 1986. This statement was produced by the World Health Organization following the first International Conference on Health Promotion meeting in Ottawa, Canada. The principles espoused by the Charter are shown in Table 20.2. It has been extremely influential over how governments and health providers think of health promotion.

The Ottawa Charter recognised that the potential to improve health on a population basis was limited by the then-prevailing health education approach. It stressed the need to work at a 'higher level' and tackle the wider determinants of health by addressing issues at the level of personal autonomy, communities and public policy.

Upstream and downstream health promotion

These terms arise from the concepts in the Ottawa Charter. Upstream refers to actions taken at a policy level to prevent disease and promote health. Downstream actions are those carried out at an individual level. As they have greater potential to reach many more people and do not require them to take any action individually, upstream actions are potentially more effective than downstream actions. Policies directed at controlling the production and availability of sugared sweets and drinks are likely to be more effective than actions by a dentist advising patients on dietary restrictions of sugar (Figure 20.2).

Table 20.2 The principles of the Ottawa Charter

• **Promoting health through public policy:** this recognises that it is necessary to reach beyond the health sector to address the determinants of health fully. Restriction on the sale of tobacco and alcohol to children is an example of a health-protecting public policy.
• **Creating a supportive environment:** this recognises the socio-geographical and environmental aspects of promoting health. Banning smoking in public places is an example of how the environment in pubs and clubs has been changed to protect bar workers from the dangers of passive smoking (breathing someone else's tobacco smoke).
• **Developing personal skills:** this involves helping individuals to develop the skills necessary to keep themselves and their families healthy. An example would be teaching young parents how to prepare and cook fresh fruit and vegetables to encourage healthy eating and reduce reliance on unhealthy pre-prepared and ultra-processed foods.
• **Strengthening community action:** this encourages local communities to come together to pool resources and knowledge to promote health – the establishment of local sports clubs would encourage physical exercise, for example.
• **Reorientating healthcare:** this involves a greater emphasis on primary care/care in communities rather than hospitals

21 Considerations in promoting oral health

Figure 21.1 Common-risk factor approach. Source: *with permission modified from Sheiham and Watt (2001).*

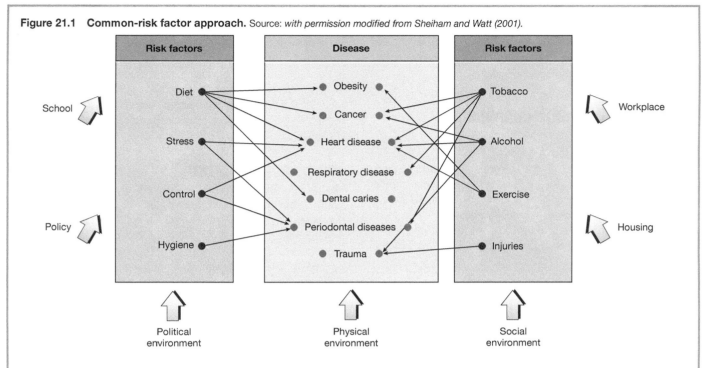

Figure 21.2 Framework for developing and evaluating complex interventions: Medical Research Council guidance (2021).
Source: *Skivington et al. (2012)/BMJ Publishing Group Limited/Public Domain CC BY 4.0.*

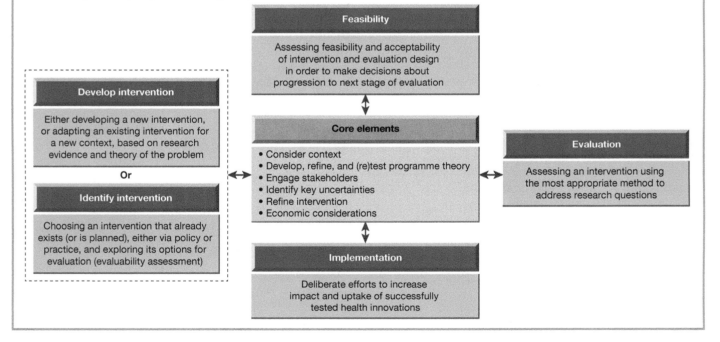

Tackling risk factors

Addressing risk factors for disease can be approached from two perspectives: a disease-centred approach and a common risk factor approach.

Disease-centred approach

In this outdated approach, the risk factor(s) for an individual disease is considered solely in relation to that one disease. This can lead to conflicting advice being given and failure to maximise the impact of preventive activities. For example, foods like cheese and potato crisps are not cariogenic, and so if health educators were to approach the prevention of dental caries purely from a dental perspective, the message that cheese is acceptable as a snack between meals might be acceptable and thus promoted. However, those concerned with the prevention of obesity and cardiovascular disease would be likely to be less happy to promote these foods as a snack.

Common risk factor approach

Here, the focus is not on a single disease but, as the name implies, on the risk factors. This approach recognises that one risk factor can contribute to more than one disease. Helping people stop smoking not only reduces the risk of developing cardiovascular disease, but oral cancer, periodontal attachment loss and any of the many other diseases in which tobacco use increases disease risk. A diagrammatic representation of the common risk factor approach is presented in Figure 21.1. This shows how alcohol is a risk factor for cancers, heart disease and trauma.

The common risk factor approach reduces the danger of individuals being given conflicting advice and maximises the health gain from adopting the advice given. Dental public health practitioners should look for opportunities to ensure that messages relevant to oral health are given when general health promotion campaigns are being planned. For example, in smoking cessation campaigns, it is important to include the effects of smoking on oral health as well as general health.

Settings approach to health promotion

In this context, a **setting** is a place or environment where groups of similar individuals meet or gather. Examples are schools, hospitals and workplaces. Sometimes, health promotion campaigns and actions are based on settings. The concept of 'health-promoting schools' has been used to ensure that schools and education authorities facilitate healthy behaviours and offer appropriate messages to children. This might involve environmental changes such as banning vending machines selling sugared drinks, the provision of water to drink in class and the promotion of fruit-only tuck shops. Educational activities would focus on health issues relevant to children and young people, such as advice on smoking, alcohol, bullying and sexual health issues.

The role of the media and technology in promoting health

Traditional media

Newspaper, magazine, billboard, radio and television advertising is occasionally used to promote health education messages. Graphic images and messages associated with smoking or the effects of not wearing a seat belt are examples. These are effective in raising awareness. However, advertising is expensive, and health bodies usually do not have an advertising budget to compete with companies advertising sugar-rich foods and drinks. Advertisements promoting cigarettes are banned in the United Kingdom. Similarly, restrictions have been implemented on advertising sugary foods and drinks during children's television programmes.

Social media

Social media – blogs, Instagram, X (formerly Twitter), Facebook, forums and message boards – are a route whereby health improvement messages can be communicated and the opinions of stakeholders gathered. Patient and public involvement (PPI) in the design and delivery of health-promoting activities is important and increases engagement and potential take-up. Social media also provides a means of disseminating messages to groups whom it might otherwise be difficult to reach, such as teenagers. Social media can also be a route where misinformation and scare stories can be easily disseminated, such as by those opposed to vaccination during the COVID-19 pandemic.

Social marketing

Social marketing uses techniques from the world of marketing to influence behaviours that benefit individuals and communities for the greater social good (rather than marketing the use of goods or services). This technique has been employed successfully in Australia to encourage the use of sun-screening products by fair-skinned individuals exposed to the fierce Antipodean sun.

Health literacy

The World Health Organization defines health literacy as 'the personal characteristics and social resources needed for individuals and communities to access, understand, appraise and use information and services to make decisions about health'.

Evaluating oral health promotion

Health promotion is about giving people control over and the chance to improve their health, but it also involves complex social and political interventions: education, facilitation and advocacy. Like with all healthcare, it is important to ensure that health promotion activities are evidence-based and achieve the desired outcome. This can be complex, given that the ultimate desired outcome – improved health, environmental or social conditions – may occur months, years or even decades after the intervention. A framework for developing and evaluating complex interventions has been published by the Medical Research Council (Figure 21.2).

The following factors should be considered when evaluating a health promotion intervention:

- **Effectiveness**: whether the aims and objectives of the intervention have been met.
- **Appropriateness**: the relevance of the intervention to needs.
- **Acceptability:** the degree to which the intervention is acceptable and carried out sensitively.
- **Efficiency:** whether time, money and other resources devoted to the programme are well spent in relation to the benefits observed.
- **Equity:** whether the programme has been delivered in relation to needs and the capacity to benefit.

22 Behaviour change I

Figure 22.1   The components of the health belief model. (Source: *After Rosenstock et al. (1988)/Springer Nature.*)

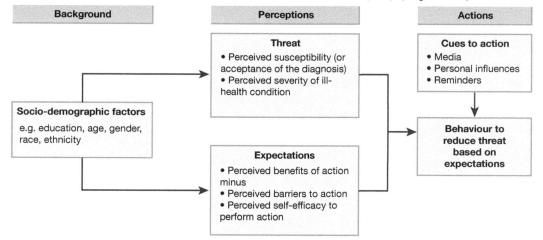

Figure 22.2   The theory of planned behaviour, which suggests that attitudes, beliefs and behavioural control are important antecedents to behaviour change. (Source: *Described by Ajzen/Elsevier.*)

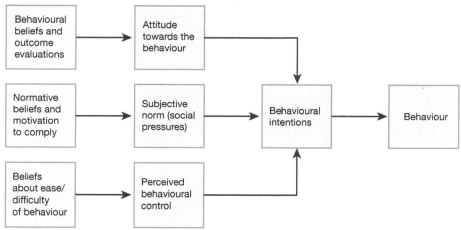

Box 22.1 The constructs underpinning the theory of planned behaviour

The Theory of Planned Behaviour comprises six constructs that collectively represent a person's actual control over their behaviour:

1 Attitude: The degree to which a person has a favourable or unfavourable evaluation of the behaviour of interest. It entails consideration of the outcomes of performing the behaviour.

2 Behavioural intention: The motivational factors that influence a given behaviour, where the stronger the intention to perform the behaviour, the more likely it is that the behaviour will be performed.

3 Subjective norms: The belief about whether most people approve or disapprove of the behaviour. It relates to a person's beliefs about whether peers and people of importance to the person think he or she should engage in the behaviour.

4 Social norms: The customary codes of behaviour in a group of people or larger cultural context. Social norms are considered normative or standard in a group of people.

5 Perceived power: The perceived presence of factors that may facilitate or impede the performance of a behaviour. Perceived power contributes to a person's perceived behavioural control over each factor.

6 Perceived behavioural control: A person's perception of the ease or difficulty of performing the behaviour of interest. Perceived behavioural control varies across situations and actions, which results in a person having varying perceptions of behavioural control depending on the situation. This construct of the theory was added later and created the shift from the Theory of Reasoned Action to the Theory of Planned Behaviour.

Dental Public Health at a Glance, Second Edition. Ivor G. Chestnutt.
© 2024 John Wiley & Sons Ltd. Published 2024 by John Wiley & Sons Ltd.

The major dental diseases are heavily influenced by lifestyle and behavioural choices. If individuals can be persuaded to change their behaviour, they can make healthy choices and avoid actions detrimental to good oral health. However, behaviour change is a complex process. Many theories of behaviour and behaviour change have been proposed, and those of most relevance to oral health are outlined here.

Knowledge, attitudes and behaviour

Knowledge → Attitudes → Behaviour

The earliest theories of behaviour change arising in the early twentieth century assumed that educating people and changing attitudes would result in behaviour change. The simplistic assumption that providing or improving knowledge via education would be sufficient to change attitudes and hence lead to sustained behaviour change has been shown to be erroneous. Psychological theories arising in the mid-twentieth century recognised that behaviour change is complicated by beliefs, ways of thinking (cognition) and environmental and social factors.

Theories of behaviour change

Three of the most common models underpinning behavior change theories are the Health belief model, the theory of planned behaviour and the trans-theoretical model.

Health belief model

The health belief model was one of the earliest health belief models and was developed in the early 1950s by social scientists at the US Public Health Service in order to understand the failure of people to adopt disease-prevention strategies or take up screening tests for early detection of disease (Figure 22.1). The model suggests that a person's likelihood of taking preventive action depends on the interaction of various beliefs:
• The perceived threat from the disease (based on the perceived susceptibility to the disease and the perceived severity or impact of the disease).
• The expectations associated with taking preventive action (based on the perceived barriers to taking action, alongside the perceived benefit of taking action in reducing the threat of a disease).

Theory of planned behaviour

The Theory of Planned Behaviour was adapted from an earlier model (the Theory of Reasoned Action). It suggests that people form positive or negative intentions to behave in a certain way bbased on their subjective norms, their perceived behavioural control and their attitude towards the behaviour. This attitude is said to be based on their belief about the likely consequences of an action and their desire to achieve those outcomes (Figure 22.2 and Box 22.1).

Trans-theoretical model

Developed by Prochaska and DiClemente in the late 1970s, this model assumes that behaviour change is evolutional in nature and occurs in stages of change through which individuals can progress. It holds that behaviours, especially habitual behaviours such as smoking, follow a series of steps through a cyclical process (Chapter 33, Figure 33.1).

NICE public health guidance on behaviour change

The National Institute of Health and Care Excellence (NICE) has issued public health guidance on behaviour change at both individual and population levels. Key findings in this guidance indicate that in promoting behaviour change, it is important to facilitate the following:
• Make people aware of outcome expectancies and help them develop accurate knowledge about the health consequences of their behaviours.
• Emphasise the personal relevance of health behaviours.
• Promote positive attitudes and feelings towards the outcomes of behaviour change.
• Promote self-efficacy by enhancing people's belief in their ability to change.
• Descriptive norms – promote the visibility of positive health behaviours in people's reference groups; that is, the groups they compare themselves to or aspire to.
• Subjective norms – enhance social approval for positive health behaviours in significant others and reference groups.
• Promote personal and moral norms – personal and moral commitments to behaviour change.
• Suggest intention formation and concrete plans – help people to form plans and goals for changing behaviours, over time and in specific contexts.
• Behavioural contracts – suggest that people share their plans and goals with others.

Locus of control

A concept that is closely related to people's health-related beliefs is their 'locus of control': the extent to which they broadly believe that their health is determined by events over which they have personal control (an internal locus of control) or events over which they have little or no control (an external locus of control).

Motivational interviewing

Motivational interviewing is a form of collaborative conversation that is designed to strengthen a person's own motivation and commitment to change. It is a person-centred style of counselling that attempts to address ambivalence about change. The process sets a specific change goal by examining the person's own reason for the change.

The ethos is that in facilitating behaviour change, the idea is not to confront the person wanting to change but to motivate them. So rather than say, 'Why don't you brush your teeth twice a day?' ask, 'What do you think would be the benefits of brushing twice a day?'

The mnemonic FRAMES is designed to help remember specific aspects of motivational interviewing:
F – provide feedback on behaviour
R – reinforce the patient's responsibility for changing behaviour
A – offer advice about changing behaviour
M – discuss a menu of options to change behaviour
E – express empathy for the patient
S – support the patient's self-efficacy (own belief in their ability to change)

It is the patient's task to say how and why they should change behaviour; the clinician's task is to elicit these arguments.

23 Behaviour change II

Figure 23.1   The components of the COM-B Model. (Source: *Michie et al. (2011) – Implementation Science 6:42 /Springer Nature / CCBY 4.0*)

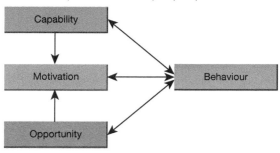

Figure 23.2   The COM-B behaviour change wheel. (Source: *Michie et al. (2011) – Implementation Science 6:42 /Springer Nature / CCBY 4.0*)

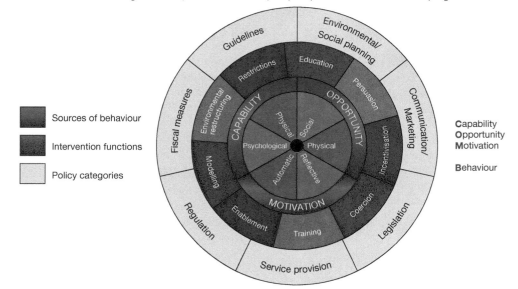

Table 23.1 The theoretical domains framework (TDF)

TDF domain	
Knowledge	Information relating to the behaviour
Skills	An ability or proficiency acquired through practice
Social/Professional role and identity	A coherent set of behaviours and displayed personal qualities of an individual in a social or work setting
Beliefs about capabilities	Acceptance of the truth, reality or validity about an ability, talent or facility
Optimism	The confidence that things will happen for the best or that the desired goals will be attained
Beliefs about consequences	Acceptance of the truth, reality or validity about outcomes of a behaviour in a given situation
Reinforcement	Increasing the probability of a response by arranging a dependent relationship, or contingency, between the response and a given stimulus
Intentions	A conscious decision to perform a behaviour or a resolve to act in a certain way
Goals	Mental representations of outcomes or end states that an individual wants to achieve
Memory, attention and decision processes	The ability to retain information, focus selectively on aspects of the environment and choose between two or more alternatives
Environmental context and resources	Any circumstance of a person's situation or environment that discourages or encourages the development of skills and abilities, independence, social competence and adaptive behaviour
Social influences	Those interpersonal processes can cause individuals to change their thoughts, feelings or behaviours
Emotion	A complex reaction pattern involving experiential, behavioural and physiological elements by which the individual attempts to deal with a personally significant matter or event
Behavioural regulation	Anything aimed at managing or changing objectively observed or measured actions

Source: *Buchanan et al. (2021); Cane et al. (2012) with permission.*

In the past century, numerous theories of behaviour change have been proposed by psychologists, educationalists, and other related disciplines. Some of the most commonly referred to are outlined in Chapter 22. Many of these theories contain common elements. Work has been undertaken to identify and combine the most important elements into a framework. The idea is that this framework or model can be used by those designing behaviour change interventions to devise programmes that have the best chance of achieving the desired aim of sustained behaviour change.

The framework/model is the closely related **theoretical domains framework (TDF)** and the **capability opportunity motivation model** – referred to as the **COM-B model**.

Theoretical Domains Framework

The Theoretical Domains Framework (TDF) consists of 14 domains (Table 23.1). Using consensus methodology to gain agreement between experts in the field of behaviour change, these 14 domains were derived from 83 theories of behaviour change which contained 128 psychological constructs. A construct is a tool used to understand human behaviour.

Capability opportunity motivation – Behaviour (COM-B) Model

The capability opportunity motivation – behaviour (COM-B) model holds that an individual's ability to change is dependant on their **Capability** to perform the behaviour, the **Opportunity** to perform the behaviour and the **Motivation** to engage in the behaviour at a given time (Figure 23.1).

In the COM-B model, each component is broken down into two elements.

Capability includes *Psychological* aspects such as possession of the necessary knowledge and the ability to understand its application and to reason. *Physical* aspects of capability include the skills to carry out the intended change, such as dexterity and strength.

Opportunity factors are external to the individual and include *Physical factors,* which are environmental, such as access to resources and materials, or *Social factors,* which are social norms or behaviours that support or inhibit attempts at behaviour change.

Motivation comprises *Reflective* processes, such as planning and goal setting, and *Automatic* processes such as the influence of habits and emotions.

The COM_B model is most easily understood as *"individuals need to be sufficiently capable to perform the behaviour, have a suitable opportunity as well as the motivation to do it".*

The relationship between the COM-B model and the TDF is shown in Table 23.2.

Table 23.2 The COM-B Model and its relation to the theoretical domains framework (TDF)

COM-B		TDF domain
Capability	Psychological	Knowledge
		Skills
		Memory and decision processes
	Physical	Behavioural regulation
		Skills
Opportunity	Social	Social influences
	Physical	Environmental context and resources
Motivation	Reflective	Social/Professional role and identity
		Beliefs about capability
		Optimism
		Beliefs about consequences
		Intentions
		Goals
	Automatic	Social/Professional role and identity
		Optimism
		Reinforcement
		Emotion

Source: *Buchanan et al. (2021); Cane et al. (2012) with permission.*

The behaviour change wheel

Closely linked to COM-B is the behaviour change wheel (BCW) (Figure 23.2). The BCW is designed to help anyone planning a behaviour change intervention (like encouraging a less cariogenic diet) to think about the various elements of behaviour change summarised in both the COM-B model and the related Theoretical Domains Framework.

The three concentric segments in the BCW capture sources of behaviour, intervention functions and policy categories, respectively, from inner to outer.

In designing a behaviour change intervention, it is necessary to think about how the intervention might be influenced by the components of the COM-B model. How do the factors identified in COM-B and the BCW need to be accounted for in designing the intervention? Which of these proximal determinants of behaviour change can be used to facilitate and make behaviour change the likely outcome?

In other words, what changes have to be made, what things have to be accounted for or overcome or put in place in order that there is the greatest chance of helping patients change behaviour and sustain that change.

To date, only a limited number of oral health-related behaviour change interventions have explicitly used the COM-B/BCW wheel.

24 Strategies for improving oral health in populations

Figure 24.1   Approaches to tackling oral health improvement. (a) High-risk individuals. (b) Whole population. (c) High-risk population. (d) Proportionate universalism

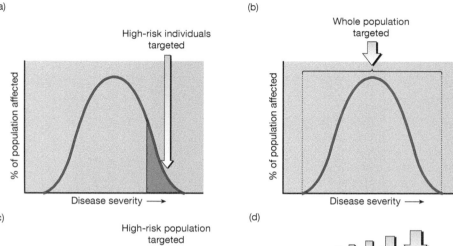

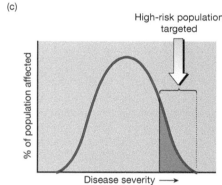

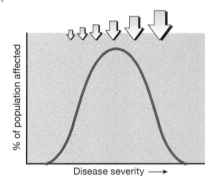

Proportionate universalism: targeted in proportion to disease severity

Figure 24.2   Example of an oral health improvement target

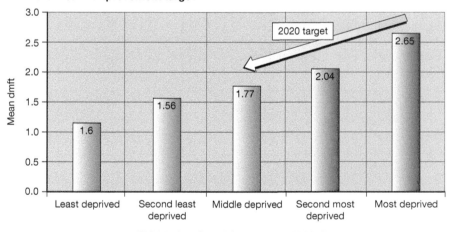

Welsh index of multiple deprivation 2008–Quintiles

Set in 2008 as part of the Welsh Child Poverty Reduction Programme, the objective is by 2020, to reduce the prevalence of dental caries in the fifth most deprived quintile of the population to that experienced by the middle deprived quintile in 2008

Dental Public Health at a Glance, Second Edition. Ivor G. Chestnutt.
© 2024 John Wiley & Sons Ltd. Published 2024 by John Wiley & Sons Ltd.

Improving population oral health can be approached in a number of ways

- High-risk individual approach
- Whole population approach
- Targeted population approach
- Proportionate universalism

High-risk individual approach

This approach to improving health involves the identification of those individuals who are at particular risk of disease and taking measures to reduce exposure to identified risk factors. This approach is applied in clinical practice on a daily basis, and it seeks to protect susceptible individuals (Figure 24.1a).

Example: A 6-year-old child attending a dental practice can be identified as at high risk for dental caries based on already having decay in their primary dentition and the dentist's knowledge of the child's family and life circumstances. The clinician would then identify the child as requiring additional preventive care, and the provision of fissure sealants, fluoride varnish and dietary counselling would be appropriate.

Whole population approach

This approach is attributed to the thinking of Geoffrey Rose, who argued that it was necessary to consider not only the determinants of disease in individuals, but also the determinants of incidence rates in different populations. This approach seeks to control the causes of incidence. In relation to dental caries, it has been argued that targeting high-risk individuals while benefiting those identified neglects the fact that the majority of new carious lesions occur in lower-risk individuals simply because there are many more of them.

Example: Advice to the whole population to 'brush your teeth twice a day with a fluoride-containing toothpaste' targets everyone and is held to have resulted in a massive shift in the distribution of dental decay in the population as a whole since the early 1970s (Figures 5.5 and 24.1b).

Targeted population approach

This approach to improving oral health is a hybrid of the high-risk and whole-population approaches. Here, the assessment of risk is not made on an individual basis, but on a population or locality basis. The correlation between dental caries and social and economic deprivation means that a much greater proportion of children resident in disadvantaged areas will experience dental decay. Population-based preventive efforts such as supervised school-based tooth-brushing programmes can be directed at these geographical localities.

Example: The Designed to Smile oral health improvement programme in Wales is an example of a targeted population approach. Here, efforts are focused on areas of social and economic deprivation in an attempt to improve oral health where disease is at its highest and by doing so address inequalities across the social spectrum (Figure 24.1c).

Proportionate universalism

Described by Marmot, this concept encourages an approach that, rather than targeting all available preventive resources at those at highest risk, proposes that preventive measures should be applied across the population in proportion to risk. This combines the advantages of all the other approaches described (Figure 24.1d).

The impact of preventive strategies on health inequalities

Setting strategies for populations with the intent of reducing inequalities in health needs careful consideration. A whole population approach, applied without appropriate care, can potentially widen health inequalities (Figure 19.3). This can occur if the preventive activity is taken up by the least deprived to a greater extent than the most deprived – which is a highly likely scenario, given that the less deprived are better placed and probably more motivated to take advantage of health improvement initiatives.

Example: In the 1970s and 1980s, before the dominance of the topical effect of fluoride in preventing dental caries was realised, fluoride tablet and drop distribution schemes were popular as a population preventive measure, the thinking being that the fluoride would be taken up by the teeth during development. Issues of how fluoride works aside, these schemes had limited impact, as it was the motivated parents, whose children were at lower risk, who were most likely to adhere to the regime of giving their children the fluoride supplements and to seek out further supplies. As a result, population-based fluoride supplement distribution schemes have long since been abandoned.

Targets in healthcare and health improvement

A target is a numerical goal often set as a policy objective. There is much debate on the merits of setting targets in healthcare. Unless they are carefully chosen, there is an argument that they have the potential to skew clinical priorities. However, politicians favour targets as a simple means of assessing the success or otherwise of the National Health Service. Perhaps the best-known example of a healthcare target in the NHS was that no one should have to wait for more than four hours before being seen in an Accident and Emergency department – a target that has proven almost impossible to meet during and following the COVID-19 pandemic (Chapter 45).

When developing health improvement strategies, it can be helpful to set a target. One example was when the Designed to Smile programme was established in Wales in 2008. This stated that by 2020, the prevalence of dental decay in 5-year-olds in the most deprived quintile should have fallen to that present in the middle deprived quintile in 2008 (thereby reducing inequalities in oral health; Figure 24.2). This target was achieved in 2015/2016.

Assessing disease risk

In the past three decades, much research has been carried out to develop risk assessment tools to determine individual susceptibility to developing oral disease. The multifactorial nature of dental caries, periodontal disease and oral cancer means that there has been limited success in the development of a single diagnostic risk assessment test. In assessing dental caries risk, the two most significant risk indicators for future caries development in children have been previous experience with dental caries and the subjective opinion of the treating clinician. General risk assessment tools such as the **assessment of clinical oral risks and needs (ACORN)** have been developed for use with individual patients in general dental practice.

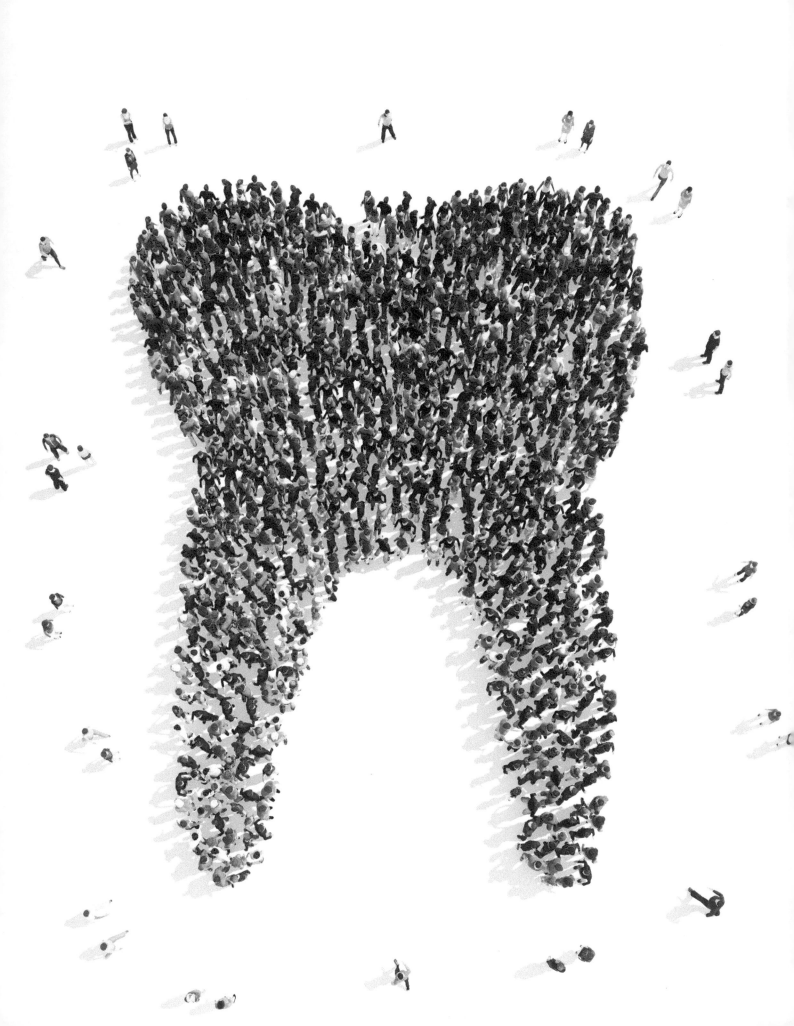

Fluoride and oral health

Part 5

Chapters

25 Strategies for the delivery of fluoride in the prevention of dental caries

Figure 25.1 Fluoride in the plaque biofilm inhibits demineralisation and promotes remineralisation of the hydroxyapatite crystals that form the tooth enamel

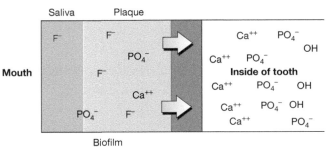

Figure 25.2 (a) Fluoride concentration in biofilm – sufficient to have caries protective effect, (b) Fluoride concentration in biofilm – exposure insufficient to have a clinically beneficial effect

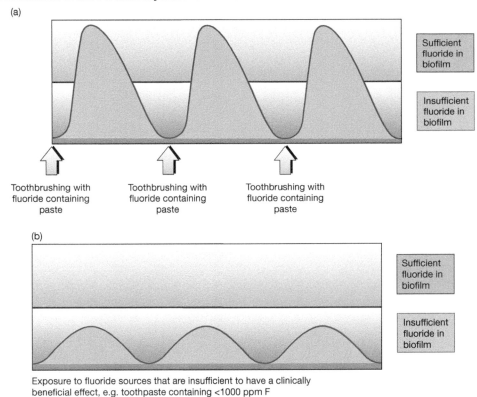

(a)

Sufficient fluoride in biofilm

Insufficient fluoride in biofilm

Toothbrushing with fluoride containing paste

Toothbrushing with fluoride containing paste

Toothbrushing with fluoride containing paste

(b)

Sufficient fluoride in biofilm

Insufficient fluoride in biofilm

Exposure to fluoride sources that are insufficient to have a clinically beneficial effect, e.g. toothpaste containing <1000 ppm F

Figure 25.3 Fluoride strategies

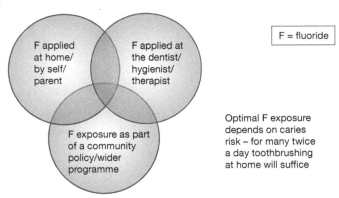

F applied at home/ by self/ parent

F applied at the dentist/ hygienist/ therapist

F = fluoride

F exposure as part of a community policy/wider programme

Optimal F exposure depends on caries risk – for many twice a day toothbrushing at home will suffice

Dental Public Health at a Glance, Second Edition. Ivor G. Chestnutt.
© 2024 John Wiley & Sons Ltd. Published 2024 by John Wiley & Sons Ltd.

How fluoride acts to prevent dental caries

To understand how fluoride can be used to prevent dental caries at a population level, it is necessary to review how fluoride works to prevent dental decay at an anatomical and biochemical level. Dental enamel is composed in the main of calcium and phosphate ions in a crystalline structure called hydroxyapatite. When the pH of the fluid within the plaque biofilm immediately adjacent to the tooth falls due to bacterial acids derived from the fermentation of dietary carbohydrates, calcium and phosphate ions are lost from the enamel crystals. Initially, this happens below the surface in the depths of the enamel prisms, as the acid acts on the porous areas between the enamel prisms that are vulnerable to acid attack. The earliest visible sign of this process is a 'white spot' enamel lesion. Unchecked, this process proceeds until a cavity develops.

From the discovery of the anticariogenic potential of fluoride in the early twentieth century until the beginning of the 1980s, it was thought that the main mechanism of action of fluoride in the prevention of dental caries depended on its incorporation into the dental enamel during tooth development pre-eruption – the systemic effect. The substitution of the hydroxyl ions in the hydroxyapatite crystals with a fluoride ion results in fluorapatite. This is more resistant to breakdown when subject to attack by acids derived from the fermentation of sugar by cariogenic bacteria once the tooth erupts into the mouth.

However, it is now understood that while the systemic effect occurs, the main mechanism of action of fluoride is its effect in encouraging the net uptake of calcium and fluoride ions at the tooth surface post-eruption – the topical effect. The presence of fluoride ions in the plaque fluid or biofilm that covers the tooth surface acts to drive calcium and phosphate into the tooth – remineralisation (Figure 25.1). Fluoride works to inhibit demineralisation at the crystal surfaces inside the tooth and to enhance the remineralisation at the crystal surfaces – the resulting remineralised layer is very resistant to subsequent acid attacks.

Research has also shown that fluoride inhibits sugar metabolism by plaque bacteria, but this effect is likely to be of limited clinical significance. It is the topical effect that is most important.

Fluoride in the plaque biofilm

In order that fluoride can exert this topical effect, it needs to be present in the plaque biofilm at a sufficient level to facilitate remineralisation and prevent demineralisation. Regular exposure to fluoride at recurring intervals helps maintain a level of fluoride that is sufficiently high to have an anticariogenic or cariostatic effect (Figure 25.2a). Exposure to sources of fluoride that contain an insufficiently high concentration or are used insufficiently frequently results in a lack of caries protection (Figure 25.2b).

Mechanisms for delivering fluoride

Fluoride can be made available in three main ways: via vehicles that patients apply themselves, via agents applied by dental professionals, via community fluoridation schemes (Table 25.1).

Table 25.1 Mechanisms for the delivery of fluoride as a caries-preventive agent

Applied by patient or their parent	Applied by a dental professional: dentist, hygienist or therapist (in the UK, dental nurses who have undergone additional training can apply fluoride varnish)	Community fluoridation schemes
Toothpaste (dentifrices)	Varnish	Water
Mouthwash	Gels	Milk
Tablets and drops	Indirectly via restorative materials, e.g. glass ionomer cement	Salt

Note: *Evidence for the effectiveness of these different ways of delivering fluoride is discussed in Chapters 26–28.*

Developing a fluoride strategy

Public health professionals, in designing strategies to protect and improve oral health, need to think about how different sources of fluoride may combine to provide a level of protection relative to the risk of different population groups to provide optimal exposure to fluoride for each individual in the population (Figure 25.3). This is dictated by caries risk.

For those who maintain good oral hygiene and who do not consume a diet that exposes them to fermentable carbohydrates in excess quantity or frequency, twice-daily brushing with a toothpaste that contains at least 1000 parts per million (ppm) fluoride will provide adequate fluoride exposure. For those at greater risk of dental caries, additional fluoride supplementation in the form of fluoride mouthwashes (e.g. when wearing a fixed orthodontic appliance) or fluoride varnish applied by a member of the dental team (e.g. when multiple early caries lesions are detected during a clinical examination) may be required. If using a fluoride mouthwash, this should be used at different times of the day to toothbrushing to maintain a sufficient background level of fluoride in the biofilm.

Community fluoridation schemes have one major advantage over professionally or self-applied fluoride – they do not require any active involvement on the part of the individual at risk. This is fortuitous, as those at greatest risk of dental caries (lower social and economic classes) are also those least likely to take active steps to use fluoride regularly or to maintain a low-sugar diet.

Exposure to excess fluoride and dental fluorosis

Exposure to excess fluoride during the period of tooth formation risks interfering with the secretion and maturation of the dental enamel on the tooth crown. Excess levels of fluoride in the body at this time can disrupt the functioning of ameloblasts. As a result, on eruption, teeth can have defects in the enamel structure – fluorosis. These range from mild white spots (hypomineralisation), which are barely noticeable unless the tooth is dried and examined carefully, to structural defects in the enamel, which appear as brownish-yellow pits (hypoplasia). Fluorosis can be distinguished from other defects of dental enamel as it has a symmetrical distribution about the midline.

26 Toothpaste

Table 26.1 Factors affecting the clinical effectiveness of toothpaste in preventing dental caries

Factor	Notes
Presence of fluoride-containing toothpaste versus non-fluoride paste	A systematic review of 70 studies (involving 42,300 children) reported that when tested against a non-fluoride control, fluoride toothpaste demonstrated a pooled prevented fraction of 24% DMFS. The 95% confidence interval was 21–28% with $P < 0.0001$. This means that fluoride toothpaste will reduce caries experience by about one-quarter. A number needed to treat analysis showed that 1.6 children need to brush with a fluoride toothpaste to prevent one DMFS in populations with a caries increment of 2.6 DMFS per year. In populations with a caries increment of 1.1 DMFS per year, 3.7 children need to brush to avoid one DMFS.
Fluoride concentration	A systematic review demonstrated that toothpastes containing a fluoride concentration of 550 parts per million (ppm) F were no more effective than a non-fluoride control. Toothpastes between 1000 and 1250 ppm F have a prevented fraction of 23%, while those containing between 2400 and 2800 ppm F prevented 36% more caries than the non-fluoride control.
Volume of toothpaste	The amount of toothpaste used by young children should be carefully controlled to avoid excess exposure to fluoride during the period of tooth formation and thereby reduce the risk of dental fluorosis. Young children should not be allowed to eat toothpaste or lick the tube. Like all medicines, toothpaste should be stored safely out of the reach of children. **Children aged up to 3 yr** Use no more than a thin smear of toothpaste (a thin film of paste covering less than three-quarters of the brush). The toothpaste should contain no less than 1000 ppm F. **Children aged 3–6 yr** Use a pea-sized amount of toothpaste containing 1350–1500 ppm F.
Method of rinsing	In clinical trials where children were asked how they rinsed their mouth after brushing, those who rinsed from a beaker had more caries than those who rinsed using less water. It is important not to rinse after brushing for maximal effect, as this washes the fluoride down the sink, and the topical effect is lost. However, it is important that children do not swallow toothpaste, especially in the period when the teeth are developing. Hence the message: **SPIT – DON'T RINSE**.
Frequency of tooth brushing	Those who brush at least twice a day experience significantly less caries than those who brush once a day or less.
Time spent brushing	There is no good evidence on the optimal time to spend brushing. Spending sufficient time to remove plaque and biofilm from difficult-to-reach areas seems sensible. Two minutes is often suggested as the optimum time.
Morning or night-time brushing	Brushing the last thing at night and not eating or drinking afterwards is important in ensuring that a good intraoral fluoride reservoir is available overnight.
Brush before or after breakfast	There is a concern that brushing immediately after eating, especially if an acidic drink has been consumed, risks removing calcium and phosphate from the fluid adjacent to the tooth surface. The alternative view is that not brushing after breakfast leaves the oral cavity deficient in fluoride.
Starting tooth brushing	Parents should be encouraged to brush their child's teeth with a smear of toothpaste containing 1000 ppm F from when the teeth first erupt.
Powered versus manual toothbrush	There is evidence of a difference in the effectiveness of powered versus manual tooth brushing. However, both are likely to be equally effective in increasing the concentration of intraoral fluoride.

History

Powders and potions for cleaning teeth date back to ancient civilisations. Over the centuries, many different ingredients have been used, such as soot, chalk, crushed eggshells and tree bark. These medicaments had no therapeutic effect other than perhaps freshening the mouth if combined with herbs and oils.

Modern toothpaste contain a combination of 'active ingredients' aimed at simultaneously combating a range of oral conditions and, in recent years, have focused on the cosmetic as well as the therapeutic benefits of toothpaste.

Fluoride-containing toothpaste

The widespread availability of fluoride-containing toothpaste from the 1970s onwards is thought to have played a major role in the improvement in oral health seen in most developed countries. Various forms of fluoride have been incorporated into toothpaste over the years. The most common formulations contain either sodium fluoride, sodium monofluorophosphate or a combination of both. It is accepted that to be effective, fluoride toothpaste should contain a minimum of 1000 parts per million (ppm) F. In the United Kingdom, the maximum concentration of fluoride that can be sold directly to the public is 1500 ppm F. Fluoride toothpaste containing 2800 ppm F, and 5000 ppm F are available on prescription for use by adolescents and adults at particularly high caries risk, on the advice of a dental professional. The cost of high-dose fluoride toothpastes means that they should be used to control and reduce caries risk, to reduce such risk to a level that can be managed by a 1500 ppm F product.

Factors that influence the clinical effectiveness of toothpaste in preventing dental caries are summarised in Table 26.1.

The safety of fluoride

Excess consumption of fluoride during the period of tooth formation can result in fluorosis. Steps to avoid exposure in young children are described in Table 26.1.

Acute toxicity can occur if someone is exposed to levels of fluoride in excess of 5 mg F/kg body weight. For a child weighing 10 kg, ingestion of 50 mg F will probably constitute a toxic dose. This equates to 50 g of a 1000 ppm F toothpaste or 33.3 g of a 1500 ppm F toothpaste.

In the event of a suspected acute overdose, if the exposure is <5 mg/kg body weight, drink large volumes of milk and seek medical advice. If exposure is >5 mg/kg body weight, refer the individual to the hospital for gastric lavage without delay.

Other active ingredients in toothpaste

In addition to fluoride, toothpastes can contain other active ingredients aimed at improving oral health (Table 26.2).

Table 26.2 Ingredients in toothpaste

Condition against which toothpaste is directed	Active ingredient(s)	Notes
Dental caries	Fluoride	The most common therapeutic agent in toothpastes.
Dental caries	Arginine and calcium salts	Studies suggest that the addition of arginine and calcium salts to fluoride toothpaste may enhance its anticaries effect, possibly by affecting the pH of the plaque biofilm
Periodontal disease	Antimicrobial agents, e.g. Chlorhexidine gluconate	Designed to have antimicrobial effects on periodontopathic organisms
Oral malodour	Antimicrobial agents, e.g. Chlorhexidine gluconate	
Calculus	Zinc citrate, pyrophosphate	Toothpastes containing these ingredients have been shown to slow down the accumulation of supra-gingival calculus
Enamel repair	Calcium silicate and sodium phosphate	Claimed to regenerate enamel through the action of calcium silicate and sodium phosphate interacting with hydroxyapatite
Erosion	Fluoride	High-dose fluoride toothpaste may be useful in combating dental erosion
Dentine sensitivity	Potassium chloride, arginine, strontium chloride, potassium nitrate, stannous fluoride	It can be helpful when dentine sensitivity is acute
Tooth discolouration	Low-dose peroxide, sodium bicarbonate, microparticles/optical brighteners, charcoal	Tooth-whitening toothpastes are currently very popular. It may have an abrasive or chemical action or both. While they may remove extrinsic staining, they do not affect intrinsic staining. Another method for whitening is the use of a film that coats the teeth to provide an optic whitening effect. Blue covarine is a typical optic brightening ingredient, though more recently, the trend has turned towards purple toothpastes. Both aim to cancel out yellow tones due to colour science (complementary colours neutralise each other, and blue/purple and yellow are complementary). Charcoal toothpastes have recently been popular but there is very limited evidence of their effectiveness in whitening teeth. These might have an immediate whitening effect but won't last as saliva washes away most paste quite rapidly.
Other ingredients in toothpaste		
	Abrasive – Hydrated silica, mica and calcium carbonate	To provide efficient cleaning. In times past, 'smokers' toothpaste' had abrasives that could result in significant tooth-surface loss. However, *in vitro* tests suggest that the abrasives in modern toothpastes are such that it would take many years to remove 1 mm of tooth structure.
	Humectants and binders	These serve to stop the toothpaste from drying out and combine the ingredients.
	Detergents and surfactants	The detergents help loosen debris and make the toothpaste foam.
	Flavours, preservatives and colouring	

27 Water fluoridation

Table 27.1 Milestones in the history of water fluoridation

Date	Milestone
1915	**Colorado stain and caries risk**. Fredrick McKay, a public health dentist in Colorado, USA, reported a developmental defect affecting the teeth of local residents. This was shown to be due to excess fluoride in the drinking water. Natural fluoridation occurs due to the local geology. Fluoride is absorbed by water flowing over fluoride-rich rocks and soil on its way to the storage reservoir/aquifer. Crucially, McKay also observed that those affected by fluorosis were less likely to experience dental decay.
1933	**Dean and optimal fluoridation**. Another American public health dentist, Trendly Dean, reported that when fluoride was present at the level of one part per million (1 ppm), the prevalence of dental caries was still low, while fluorosis was also mild.
1945	**The first artificial fluoridation study**. Evidence from the observational studies of McKay, Dean and others in the first half of the twentieth century led to the hypothesis that adding fluoride to the public water supply could act as a caries-preventive measure. The first such study involved three cities in the US state of Michigan. Fluoride was added to the water supply of the town of Grand Rapids (where the water supply was deficient in fluoride). The city of Muskegon (also lacking fluoride) acted as a control, while the town of Aurora, which was naturally fluoridated, acted as a positive control. After 6.5 years, the prevalence of dental caries in Grand Rapids had fallen by 50%, at which time Muskegon also fluoridated its water supply.
1950	The Medical Research Council's UK studies.
1980	**The Strathclyde Fluoridation Case**. This lengthy legal case established that the only impediment to water fluoridation in Scotland at the time was the lack of legal authority to do so on the part of Strathclyde Council. Representations on the idea of 'mass medication' and the adverse health effects of fluoride were rejected by the court.
1985	**The 1985 Water (Fluoridation) Act**. This stated: 'When requested by a health authority, the water supplier *may*, while the application remains in force, increase the fluoride content of the water supplied by them within that area.' The word 'may' in this legislation was a crucial impediment to implementing fluoridation schemes in the United Kingdom. Following privatisation of the water industry, water companies interpreted the legislation as permissive rather than obligatory. Concerns over who would be responsible for indemnity in the event of an accident also hindered the implementation of fluoridation.
2000	**The York Review**. This UK government-commissioned systematic review examined the clinical effectiveness and safety of water fluoridation. It established that fluoridation did reduce the prevalence of dental caries. The only adverse outcome was an increased prevalence of fluorosis in fluoridated areas. There was no credible evidence that fluoridation had an adverse impact on general health.
2002	**Medical Research Council Review**. This review suggested the need for research on the public's perception of fluorosis, trends on exposure to fluoride in an era of widespread fluoride toothpaste use and the effects of fluoridation on the oral health of adults.
2003	**Water Act 2003 Section 58 (Fluoridation of Water Supplies)**. This clarified indemnity issues (the government would be responsible) and removed water companies' veto, saying they had to fluoridate if asked to by the Strategic Health Authorities. However, Health Authorities were, as a result of this legislation, required to consult with the local population prior to implementation of a new water-fluoridation scheme.
2007	**Australian National Health and Medical Research Council**. This review concluded that 'the existing body of evidence strongly suggests that fluoridation is beneficial for reducing dental caries'.
2015	**Cochrane Review**. Raised doubts about the quality and age of the evidence supporting fluoridation.
2022	**Health and Care Bill: water fluoridation**. Gave the Secretary of State the power to directly introduce, vary or terminate water fluoridation schemes. Prior to this the responsibility lay with local authorities. The Bill also transfered the requirement from local authorities to the Secretary of State to consult water supply companies on whether any fluoridation scheme variation or termination to existing schemes are operable and efficient, prior to undertaking any public consultation on schemes.

*F*luoridation = the adjustment of the level of fluoride in public water supplies with the intention of preventing dental caries.

The addition of fluoride to the public water supply to prevent dental caries has been practised for nearly 70 years. Key milestones in the fluoridation story are highlighted in Table 27.1. The Centers for Disease Control (CDC) in America have described water fluoridation as one of the twentieth century's ten great public health achievements.

The global epidemiology of water fluoridation

According to the British Fluoridation Society, some 337 million people worldwide receive artificially fluoridated water. A further 18 million drink water in which fluoride is naturally present at an optimal level to prevent dental caries. Fluoridation is widespread in the United States. Around 208 million Americans receive optimally fluoridated water – about 74% of the population. Of the 50 largest American cities, 47 have optimally fluoridated water. In Canada, population coverage is estimated at 44%. Fluoridation schemes are widespread in South America (Brazil 41%, Chile 65%), and many countries in Asia are extensively fluoridated – Singapore (100%), Hong Kong (100%) and Malaysia (75%). Fluoridation is very much less widespread in Europe. Only Spain (11%), the Republic of Ireland (73%), Serbia (3%) and England (10%) fluoridate their water supplies. The epidemiology of fluoridation in the United Kingdom is discussed in Box 27.1.

The effectiveness of water fluoridation

Three systematic reviews have investigated the clinical effectiveness of water fluoridation. The York Review (2000) concluded that the best available evidence suggested that fluoridation of drinking water supplies reduced caries prevalence, both as measured by the proportion of the population who are caries-free and by the mean change in the number of decayed missing and filled teeth. Among 5- to 15-year-olds, water fluoridation reduced the number of caries-affected teeth by, on average, 2.25 teeth per child. This equates to an overall reduction in tooth decay of about 40%. The percentage of children free from decay in fluoridated areas was, on average, 14.6% higher than in comparable non-fluoridated areas. That review was, however, conducted more than 20 years ago, and the evidence reviewed was much older and deemed to be of limited quality. A 2015 Cochrane review noted the lack of contemporary evidence for the effectiveness of fluoridation – important given the now lower prevalence of dental caries than in decades past.

A 2022 study of water fluoridation carried out in Cumbria, England, concluded that the impact of water fluoridation was much smaller than previous studies have reported. The evidence, after adjusting for deprivation, age and sex, with an adjusted odds ratio of 0.74 (95% confidence interval 0.56–0.98), suggested that water fluoridation was likely to have a modest beneficial effect. There was insufficient evidence of a difference in the presence of decay in children in a cohort aged 5–11 years of age ($n = 1192$), with 19.1% of children in the intervention group having decay into dentine, compared with 21.9% of children in the control group (adjusted odds ratio 0.80, 95% confidence interval 0.58–1.09). There was also no significant difference in the performance of water fluoridation on caries experience across deprivation quintiles.

Recommended concentration of fluoride in water supplies

An Australian review stated that water should be fluoridated at a level between 0.6 and 1.1 ppm, depending on climate, to balance the reduction of dental caries and the occurrence of dental fluorosis. Traditionally, water fluoridation has been implemented at a concentration of 1 ppm F. Concerns over fluorosis and fluoride availability from other sources, such as toothpastes have led to a reduction to 0.5–0.8 ppm F in countries where fluoridation is practised.

The ethics of water fluoridation

The ethical aspects of water fluoridation were investigated by the Nuffield Council on Bioethics. It concluded that the argument of 'a coercive intervention' should not be accepted when adding a substance to the public water supply brought a health benefit. The acceptability of any public health policy involving the water supply should be considered in relation to:

- the balance of risks and benefits
- the potential for alternatives that rank lower on the intervention ladder to achieve the same outcome
- the role of consent where there are potential harms.

It was concluded that the most appropriate way of deciding whether to fluoridate the water supply was to rely on local democratic decision-making procedures.

Factors necessary for implementation of water fluoridation schemes

For fluoridation to be feasible, a public water supply should be present at a sufficient scale to make the scheme economically viable. Fluoride is added to the water under carefully controlled conditions during water-treatment works. The population served by these works needs to be sufficiently large, and the prevalence of caries needs to be sufficiently high to make a fluoridation scheme economically viable. Areas where the population is served by multiple small reservoirs or wells and boreholes (e.g. rural areas) are unsuitable for fluoridation. In addition to these practical considerations, political will and the necessary finance have to be present for fluoridation to be possible.

Box 27.1 Water fluoridation in the United Kingdom

In the United Kingdom, artificial fluoridation schemes operate only in England. The major fluoridation schemes operate in the West Midlands and in the North East – these schemes cover 5.8 million people. A further 0.3 million live in areas where fluoride is naturally present in the water supply at a level sufficient to prevent dental caries.

Following devolution in 1999, the position of the constituent countries of the United Kingdom has varied with respect to fluoridation. In England, the Department of Health and Social Care has, since 1998, actively pursued the implementation of new fluoridation schemes in areas of high caries prevalence – but to date without success. In Scotland, failed attempts to introduce fluoridation in the 1980s and early 1990s have led to the pursuit of alternative community fluoridation programmes in the guise of the 'Childsmile' programme. The Welsh Government accepts the benefits of water fluoridation. Still, it has no plans to implement fluoridation and, like Scotland, has opted for a school-based supervised toothbrushing programme 'Designed to Smile'.

Objections to water fluoridation

There is a small but vocal minority of individuals who are vehemently opposed to water fluoridation. Over the years, a large number of diseases, including bone fractures and various cancers, have been cited as resulting from the presence of fluoride in the public water supply. Possible adverse effects of fluoridation have been examined in systematic reviews. A meta-regression conducted as part of the York Review found no association between bone fractures and fluoridation. Similarly, no association was demonstrable between fluoridation and the incidence or mortality from any form of cancer.

Other objections raised by anti-fluoridationists include: fluoridation is a form of mass medication; fluoridation is a means of disposing of waste fluoride products from the industry; most of the water that has been fluoridated is never ingested by humans; fluoridated water poses a danger to patients undergoing kidney dialysis; and infusion of fluoride while bathing poses a health risk.

Dental fluorosis and fluoridation

While no adverse effects of fluoridation on general health have been established, it is accepted that the prevalence of dental fluorosis is increased in areas where the water supply is fluoridated. This is hardly surprising, given how the caries-preventive effect of fluoride was first discovered (Table 27.1). The degree to which this increase in fluorosis is problematic is a matter of debate.

The economics of water fluoridation

The economics of water fluoridation is related to the caries prevalence and size of the population to be served. The greater the caries prevalence and the larger the number of people served, the more effective the scheme becomes. The costs arise from the capital expenditure required to install the machinery necessary to add and monitor the fluoride. There are then the annual running costs. Savings arise from decay avoided, improvements in oral health and subsequent impact on quality of life and utility costs in not having to attend for treatment.

A 2016 rapid review carried out by the York Economics Consortium concluded that no recent robust and generalisable studies on the cost-effectiveness of water fluoridation to improve oral health in 0–5-year-olds could be identified.

In 2017, estimated costs for the implementation of a scheme by Hull City Council were between £1.6 and £2 million pounds for set up and annual running costs of £300,000 per year. Based on the most expensive estimate from a feasibility study, this fluoridation scheme would, it was estimated, generate £7.22 savings for every £1 spent for 0–5-year-olds (reduced treatment costs and time off work for parents).

Community fluoride schemes and fissure-sealant programmes

Table 28.1 Community fluoride schemes – evidence, advantages and disadvantages

Evidence	Advantages	Disadvantages
School-based supervised tooth brushing Randomised controlled trials have shown school tooth brushing to be effective Recommended by NICE oral health improvement guidelines	• Encourages tooth brushing in at-risk children • Socialises tooth brushing • Can achieve very high participation rates due to peer pressure among children in schools	• Expensive • Requires excellent cooperation with schools and education staff • Labour intensive
Fluoride varnish schemes		
Good evidence for the effectiveness of fluoride varnish when used on an individual basis in clinic	• It can be targeted at high-risk children • Do not require clinics to deliver • Can be delivered by trained dental nurses	• Require access to at-risk children • Do not necessarily encourage the uptake of tooth brushing in non-tooth-brushers
Fluoride tablets and drop distribution schemes		
Limited evidence of effectiveness at current rates of caries prevalence	• None	• Least likely to be taken up by parents of children at greatest risk • Overenthusiastic use risks overdose and fluorosis • Do not socialise routine oral hygiene behaviours – medicalises dental caries • Rely on an outdated understanding of anticaries effects of fluoride
Fluoride mouth-rinsing programmes		
Evidence of effectiveness comes mainly from the USA, where school mouth-rinse programmes have operated for many years. Suggests more effective in areas of high caries prevalence.	• It can be carried out with relatively limited disruption to school activities • It can be targeted at high-risk children	• It cannot be used in children aged <8 years
Fluoride in milk		
Evidence of effectiveness is outdated or from countries where caries prevalence is much greater than is currently the case in the UK	• There are alternatives such as fluoride varnish schemes or supervised school tooth brushing	• Relies on a school milk programme being present • Unclear whether fluoride is present at a sufficient concentration to have a beneficial effect – may simply add to background levels of fluoride without beneficial therapeutic effect
Fluoridated salt		
Evidence is old and from a time when the caries prevalence was much higher than that currently prevailing	• None – an outdated concept that has no relevance to current dental public health practice	• General public health messages are to reduce salt intake • Cannot easily be targeted to at-risk groups • Issue of whether the fluoride is present at a sufficient concentration intraorally

In the absence of water fluoridation, alternative means of increasing the contact of teeth with fluoride have been devised. Each has advantages and disadvantages (Table 28.1).

National Institute for Health and Care Excellence (NICE) guidelines on oral health improvement

The Health and Social Care Act (2012) transferred responsibility for oral health improvement programmes in England from the National Health Service to local authorities. NICE has issued guidance to local authorities on how to improve oral health in at-risk groups. This guidance supplement is meant to be used in conjunction with Delivering Better Oral Health (DBOH) – An Evidence-Based Toolkit for Prevention. Issued jointly by the Department of Health and Social Care, the Welsh Government, the Department of Health Northern Ireland, Public Health England, NHS England and NHS Improvement, and with the support of the British Association for the Study of Community Dentistry, DBOH deals mainly with improving oral health at an individual level, while the NICE guidance deals with populations or high-risk groups within the general population (Chapter 24).

School-based supervised tooth brushing

Supervised tooth brushing in schools has been used as an alternative to water fluoridation in some countries. The 'Childsmile' programme in Scotland takes a whole-population approach. In contrast, the 'Designed to Smile' programme in Wales takes a targeted-population approach, whereby the programme is directed at those deemed at greatest risk.

Fluoride varnish programmes

Fluoride varnish programmes have been introduced in areas of high dental need. Systematic reviews have shown that the application of fluoride varnish two to four times per year has a caries-preventive effect. NICE guidelines recommend this approach for children in nursery school aged three and over in areas of high caries prevalence. The most commonly used fluoride varnish contains fluoride at a concentration of 22,600 ppm F.

Fluoride tablet and drop distribution schemes

In the 1970s and 1980s, fluoride tablet and drop distribution schemes were popular in the United Kingdom. This was when the systemic effect of fluoride (incorporation of fluoride into the tooth enamel during mineralisation) was thought to be the mechanism whereby fluoride increased resistance to bacterial acids. A changed understanding of how fluoride exerts its caries-protective effects (topical), plus poor compliance by the parents of those children at greatest risk, have led to the abandonment of these schemes.

Fluoride mouth-rinsing programmes

Weekly mouth-rinsing programmes with a 0.2% NaF (sodium fluoride) solution were once very common in the United States. There are no school-based mouth-rinsing programmes in the United Kingdom, and it is not recommended as a community fluoride scheme. Daily mouth rinsing on an individual basis with a fluoride rinse containing 0.05% NaF is recommended for individuals at high risk of caries as a supplement to twice-daily tooth brushing. Mouthwashes are not recommended for children under eight years old. To maximise intraoral fluoride concentration, mouthwashes should be used at a different time of the day from tooth brushing.

Fluoride in milk

For many years, school milk was seen as a potential means of increasing the availability of fluoride to children. Schemes have been implemented with varying degrees of success in Chile, Peru, Russia and Thailand. A large scheme in the North West of England failed to demonstrate clinical benefit. Much of the work to continue milk fluoridation has been facilitated by the Borrow Foundation. This charity has as its aim to improve oral health through the greater use of fluorides, particularly via milk and milk products. Fluoridated milk is not formally recommended in current NICE guidelines.

Fluoridated salt

The addition of fluoride to salt began in some European countries, mainly Switzerland and France, in the mid-twentieth century and claims for a caries-protective effect have been made. This concept followed the addition of iodine to salt to combat goitre. Only 10% of salt intake is added by individuals to their food – the vast majority of salt is added to food during the manufacturing process. Attempts have been made to persuade bakers to use fluoridated salt in bread making. However, given the general health message about reducing the overall salt intake to protect cardiovascular health, fluoridated salt is no longer regarded as a realistic oral health protection measure in the United Kingdom.

Fluoride gels and foams

Fluoride gels and foams applied in individual trays were used in the past. However, these were only ever suitable for use on an individual patient basis in a dental clinic. They have largely been superseded by fluoride varnish.

Fissure-sealant programmes

In addition to community fluoride programmes, school-based fissure-sealant programmes have been promoted. These aim to deal with dental caries occurring on the occlusal surface of the first permanent molar teeth. The majority (80%) of tooth decay in teenagers is to be found on the occlusal surfaces of first permanent molars.

Fissure sealants are Bis-GMA (bisphenol A-glycidyl methacrylate) based materials attached to the pit and fissure surface of the teeth using acid-etch technology. They work by providing a physical barrier to the accumulation of a cariogenic plaque biofilm in the depths of the crevices, thereby reducing caries susceptibility. For maximal effectiveness, they should be applied shortly after the teeth erupt (when they are particularly caries susceptible). They should be maintained and replaced if they are lost or become defective.

A systematic review has shown that concerns about decay progression under sealants are unfounded. This means that unless there is clear evidence that the caries process has progressed into the dentine, occlusal surfaces can be sealed.

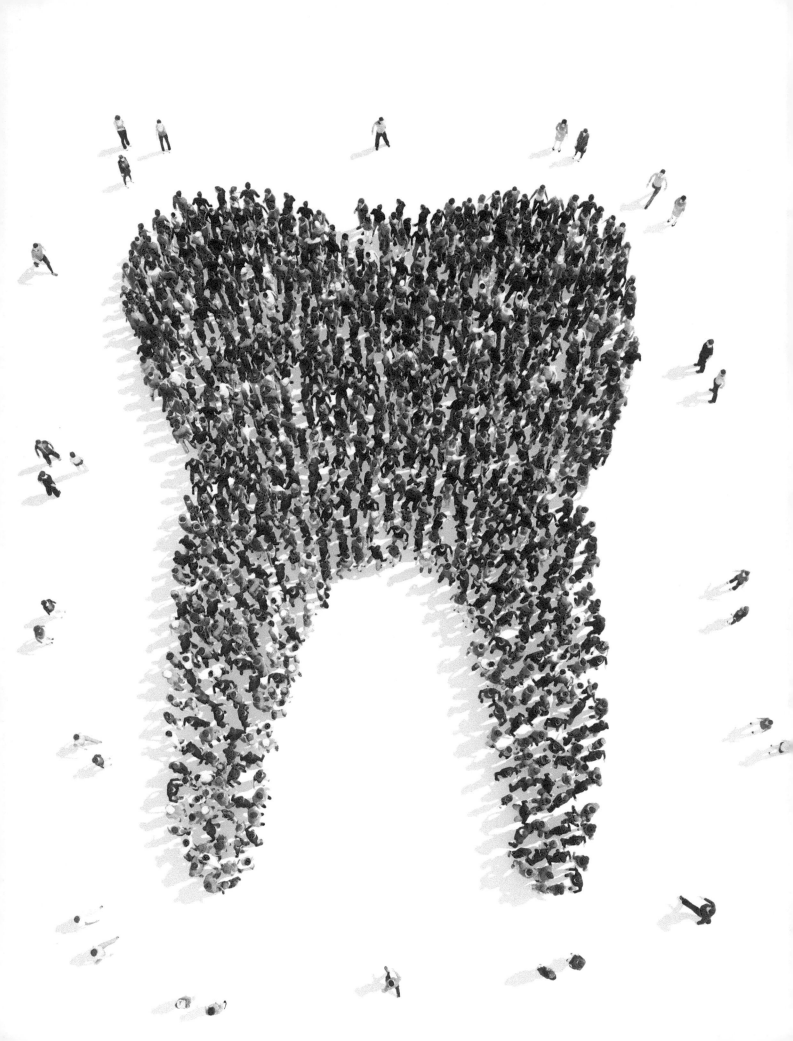

Diet and oral health

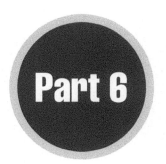

Part 6

Chapters

29 Diet and oral health

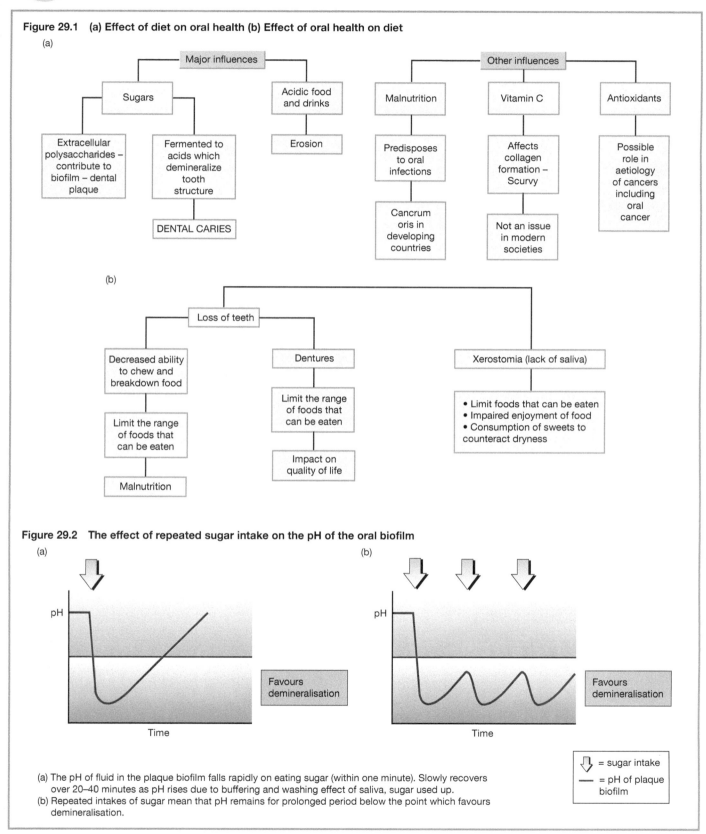

Figure 29.1 **(a) Effect of diet on oral health (b) Effect of oral health on diet**

(a)

Major influences

Sugars

Extracellular polysaccharides – contribute to biofilm – dental plaque

Fermented to acids which demineralize tooth structure

DENTAL CARIES

Acidic food and drinks

Erosion

Other influences

Malnutrition

Predisposes to oral infections

Cancrum oris in developing countries

Vitamin C

Affects collagen formation – Scurvy

Not an issue in modern societies

Antioxidants

Possible role in aetiology of cancers including oral cancer

(b)

Loss of teeth

Decreased ability to chew and breakdown food

Limit the range of foods that can be eaten

Malnutrition

Dentures

Limit the range of foods that can be eaten

Impact on quality of life

Xerostomia (lack of saliva)

- Limit foods that can be eaten
- Impaired enjoyment of food
- Consumption of sweets to counteract dryness

Figure 29.2 **The effect of repeated sugar intake on the pH of the oral biofilm**

(a)

pH

Favours demineralisation

Time

(b)

pH

Favours demineralisation

Time

⬇ = sugar intake
— = pH of plaque biofilm

(a) The pH of fluid in the plaque biofilm falls rapidly on eating sugar (within one minute). Slowly recovers over 20–40 minutes as pH rises due to buffering and washing effect of saliva, sugar used up.
(b) Repeated intakes of sugar mean that pH remains for prolonged period below the point which favours demineralisation.

Dental Public Health at a Glance, Second Edition. Ivor G. Chestnutt.
© 2024 John Wiley & Sons Ltd. Published 2024 by John Wiley & Sons Ltd.

Diet and health

A good diet and adequate nutrition are essential for health. Poor diet is a key risk factor for many chronic diseases, including cardiovascular disease, diabetes, cancers, osteoporosis, gastrointestinal disorders and dental caries. The sedentary lifestyle of modern populations, coupled with the ease of access to energy-rich and ultra-processed food and drink, has led to an increasing proportion of the population being overweight or obese. The relationship between diet and oral health works in two ways. Diet is an important predisposing risk factor for oral disease, most notably dental caries. Conversely, oral health can impact diet and nutrition (Figures 29.1a, b).

A common risk factor approach to health improvement means that messages about reducing the amount and frequency of sugar consumption related to oral health also relate to general health.

Diet and dental caries

Evidence that sugar in the diet is responsible for dental caries comes from different types of studies.

- **Animal studies:** Many of the early investigations into the effect of sugar on dental caries involved the use of animals (most commonly rats).
- *In-situ* **appliance experiments:** In these experiments, enamel slabs are mounted on intraoral appliances (i.e. part dentures that clip over teeth) and are worn by volunteers (often dental students!). Sugar solutions of varying types and concentrations are applied to the slabs *ex vivo*, and the appliance is inserted and worn for varying periods. The plaque biofilm is then 'fed' with sugar. The degree of de/remineralisation of the enamel slab can be detected by the removal of the slab from the appliance and the use of microradiography.
- **Human plaque pH studies:** An in-dwelling pH electrode can be used to measure plaque pH in real-time, as acids are produced by fermentation following the ingestion of a sugar-containing solution or foodstuff. This type of study can be used to demonstrate the effect of the frequency of sugar intake. Repeated exposure to sugar replenishes the sugar supply to the bacteria in the plaque biofilm. As a result, buffers in saliva and the washing effect of saliva are negated, and the pH at the tooth surface favours the net loss of calcium and phosphate ions (demineralisation) for as long as the repeated sugar consumption continues (Figure 29.2).
- **Observational studies:** Many studies on the role of sugar and dental caries take the form of observational studies, where the relationship is examined (cross-sectional) or over a period of time (longitudinal).
- **Cross-sectional studies**
  - *Country-by-country analysis:* A significant correlation between sugar consumption per capita and caries prevalence has been shown on a country-by-country basis. Caries levels are low when total sugar consumption is less than 10 kg/person/year, but increase rapidly when sugar consumption rises above 15 kg/person/year. This is a crude measure and takes no account of the variation of sugar consumption by individuals, and it also does not account for the frequency of sugar consumption.
  - *Communities with special diets:* The prevalence of dental caries has been examined in communities with special diets that either consume excess sugar or have a sugar-restricted diet. Confectionery workers who were at liberty to consume their products have been shown to be at greater risk for dental caries, while hereditary fructose intolerance, a developmental, metabolic defect that requires a diet low in sugar, has a low caries prevalence.
  - *Longitudinal studies and serial cross-sectional before-and-after studies:* Past studies have shown changes in caries prevalence following changes in sugar availability. Wartime studies demonstrate that the prevalence of dental caries fell during the Second World War when sugar became scarce and rose again following the increased availability of sugar when hostilities ended. Further evidence comes from remote communities whose traditional diet was low in sugar, which experienced increased caries levels when introduced to sugar-rich diets. One of the most often-quoted examples is the remote Atlantic island of Tristan da Cunha, where the oral health of the population deteriorated following the establishment of an American defence base and the resultant increased availability of sugar.
- **Intervention studies:** Manipulation of diet in an experimental setting is difficult, but there are a few often-quoted studies that have attempted this relating to oral health. The famous Vipeholm study conducted in a mental hospital in Sweden in the 1950s fed patients in different wards sugar in various formats. Many criticisms can be made of that study from an experimental and particularly ethical perspective. However, data from that study have been used to demonstrate the detrimental effects of sugar when consumed frequently and in sticky retentive forms. Another example is the Turku studies in Finland, which investigated the effects of xylitol on caries de- and remineralisation.

The quality of the evidence that sugar causes dental caries

The evidence that sugar causes dental caries is incontrovertible. However, the majority of the studies referred to were conducted in the era before fluoride was widely available in communities, either in the public water supply or in toothpaste.

Breastfeeding and dental caries

Wherever possible, new mothers should be encouraged to breastfeed – the benefits to children of breastfeeding exceed those of bottle feeding. However, there have been some reports of dental caries associated with abnormal patterns of breastfeeding, where the child is allowed to feed '*ad libitum*'; that is, at will and throughout the night.

Diet and dental erosion

A diet with a high acidic content can cause erosion of the teeth. This is most commonly seen in individuals who consume large quantities of carbonated beverages, particularly those who consume acidic drinks at frequent intervals throughout the day. Erosion can also be seen in people who eat excessive quantities of acidic fruits, such as citrus fruits and green apples.

Diet and periodontal disease

Periodontal disease is not influenced by diet to any extent. Vitamin C deficiency (scurvy) affects collagen formation, but this condition is unlikely to be encountered in dental practice.

Public health aspects of dietary modification

Figure 30.1 Forest plot of the relationship between obesity and dental caries

Group by	Study name	Statistics for each study				Std diff in means and 95% CI
Dentition type		Std diff in means	Lower limit	Upper limit	P-value	
Permanent	Alm et al., 2008	0.474	−0.062	1.010	0.083	
Permanent	Gerdin et al., 2008	0.096	0.017	0.175	0.017	
Permanent	Granville-Garcia et al., 2008	−0.027	−0.282	0.228	0.836	
Permanent	Narksawat et al. 2009	−0.530	−0.809	−0.252	0.000	
Permanent	Sadeghi and Alizadch, 2007 (permanent teeth)	0.394	0.176	0.612	0.000	
Permanent	Sharma and Hedge, 2009	0.370	0.078	0.661	0.013	
Permanent	Tramini et al., 2009	0.095	−0.259	0.450	0.599	
Permanent	Willerhausen et al., 2007 (permanent teeth)	0.239	0.053	0.425	0.012	
Permanent		0.124	−0.053	0.301	0.170	
Primary	Chenetal, 1998	0.034	−0.080	0.148	0.562	
Primary	Kopycka-Kedzierawski et al., 2008 (primary teeth)	−0.123	−0.386	0.140	0.360	
Primary	Macek and Mitola, 2008	0.140	−0.038	0.319	0.124	
Primary	Oliveira et al., 2008	−0.282	−0.563	0.000	0.050	
Primary	Sadeghi and Alizadch, 2007 (primary teeth)	0.227	0.010	0.445	0.040	
Primary	Sheller et al., 2009	0.094	−0.353	0.541	0.681	
Primary	Vazquez-Nava et al., 2009	0.362	0.179	0.544	0.000	
Primary	Willerhausen et al., 2007 (primary teeth)	0.159	−0.027	0.345	0.093	
Primary		0.093	−0.033	0.220	0.149	
Overall		0.104	0.001	0.206	0.049	

−1.00 −0.50 0.00 0.50 1.00

Favours non-caries   Favours caries

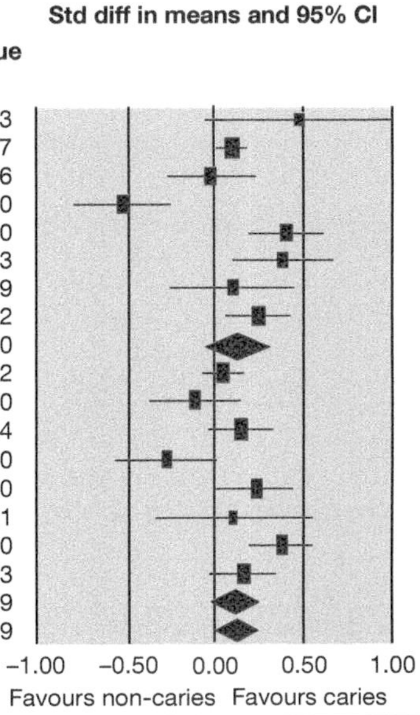

Meta analysis

A non-significant relationship is observed between obesity and dental caries in the permanent dentition (p = 0.17) and in the primary dentition (p = 0.149). A marginally significant relationship is observed when both primary and permanent dentition are combined (p = 0.049)

Table 30.1 Definitions of overweight and obesity

Children <5 yr old	
Overweight	Weight for height > ±2 standard deviations (SD) of the WHO Child Growth Standards median

School-aged children and adolescents (5–19 yr old)	
Overweight	Body Mass Index (BMI) for age > +1 SD of the WHO growth reference for school-aged children and adolescents (equivalent to BMI 25 kg/m² at 19 years)
Obese	> ±2 standard deviations of the WHO growth reference for school-aged children and adolescents (equivalent to BMI 30 kg/m² at 19 years)

Adults (>20 yr)	
Overweight	BMI > 25 kg/m²
Obese	BMI > 30 kg/m²

$$BMI = \frac{mass\,(kg)}{height\,(m)^2}$$

Source: *WHO.*

Box 30.1 Recommended sugar intake

• WHO recommends a reduced intake of free sugars throughout the lifecourse (strong recommendation)
• In both adults and children, WHO recommends reducing the intake of free sugars to less than 10% of total energy intake (strong recommendation)
• WHO suggests a further reduction of the intake of free sugars to below 5% of total energy intake (conditional recommendation)

Source: *Adapted from WHO (2015b).*

Box 30.2 Suggested actions to reduce obesity

• Multisectoral population-based policies to influence the production, marketing and consumption of healthy foods.
• Fiscal policies to increase the availability and consumption of healthy food and reduce consumption of unhealthy food.
• Promotion of breastfeeding.
• Policies and actions to reduce physical inactivity.
• Educational and social marketing campaigns focused on appropriate diet and increasing physical activity.
• Policies to reduce direct marketing and advertising of foods high in sugar and fat to children.
• Introduction of measures to create healthy eating environments.

Source: *Adapted from WHO (2015b).*

Free sugars

Free sugars are defined by the World Health Organization (WHO) as:

Monosaccharides and disaccharides added to foods and beverages by the manufacturer, cook or consumer, and sugars naturally present in honey, syrups, fruit juices and juice concentrates.

This includes sucrose and its constituent parts, fructose and glucose. Free sugars contribute to the energy density of foods. The ready availability of such foods and the consumption of them, especially sugar-sweetened beverages, can easily lead to an excess of energy intake over energy expenditure.

Recommended sugar intake

The WHO has issued guidance on the intake of sugar. Energy intake from free sugars should comprise less than 10% of energy intake and ideally would be less than 5% of total energy intake (Box 30.1).

Obesity

One of the greatest challenges to the public's health is the ever-increasing proportion of the population who are either overweight or obese. According to the WHO, more than 1 billion people worldwide are obese – 650 million adults, 340 million adolescents and 39 million children. This number is still increasing. In England, 25.3% of adults aged 18 and over were living with obesity from November 2020 to November 2021, which is an increase from 24.4% in 2019 to 2020 and 22.7% in 2015 to 2016. There is a large variation in the prevalence of adult obesity across upper-tier local authorities in England, ranging from 10.5% to 40.3%.

It is estimated that by 2050, 60% of men, 50% of women and 25% of children will be obese. Obesity has been described as 'the new smoking' and some authorities have suggested that the challenges posed by sugar in the twenty-first century equate to those posed by tobacco in the twentieth century.

Definitions of overweight and obesity are shown in Table 30.1. Suggested actions to tackle obesity are shown in Box 30.2.

Obesity and dental caries

Obesity and dental caries have in common a major dietary component in their aetiology, and in particular the consumption of sweetened beverages. However, epidemiological studies have been somewhat equivocal in demonstrating a consistent relationship between obesity and caries, some studies showing a significant association, while others fail to demonstrate such a relationship. A recent systematic review (Hayden et al. 2013) found a marginally significant association across all dentition types, but not separately for primary and permanent teeth (Figure 30.1). A further analysis by those authors using standardised measures of obesity demonstrated a more significant relationship between obesity and caries in the permanent teeth.

These findings reflect the multifactorial aetiology of both obesity and dental caries. The assumption that children who eat more are more likely to experience decay is possibly mistaken. Underweight children may well have a food intake that comprises frequent sugar-rich drinks and confectionery.

Actions to reduce sugar intake

- **Fruit tuck shops:** Many schools have banned 'tuck shops' that sell sweets and sugar-rich drinks and replaced them with shops that sell only fruit.
- **Water in schools:** In a similar vein, schools now allow children to have a bottle of water at their desks. Many insist on transparent bottles so that the contents can be clearly seen. Not only do water-in-school schemes encourage the consumption of a toothfriendly drink (i.e. water), the children are adequately hydrated.
- **Vending machines:** A ban on vending machines selling sweetened drinks has been implemented in hospitals and schools in Wales. This is a good practical example of creating a healthier environment as set out in the Ottawa Charter (Chapter 20).
- **Sweet-free checkouts:** A long-standing campaign has been conducted to persuade the major supermarkets to remove sweets and confectionery from checkouts, where placed at child's eye level, they are positioned to facilitate maximum 'pester power' at the end of a shopping trip. This campaign has met with partial success in that most supermarkets now offer at least some sweet-free check-outs.
- **Advertising directed at children:** Previous research has demonstrated that a significantly greater proportion of television advertisements during children's television time in the late afternoon was for foods and drinks than was the case at prime time during the evening. Advertisements for sugar-rich cereals were particularly common. Recent changes to advertising regulations have placed greater restrictions on how sugar-rich products are targeted at children.

Sugar substitutes

Food manufacturers have explored alternatives to sucrose and fructose as sweetening agents in 'diet' or 'light' drinks, including saccharine, aspartame and xylitol. As these agents are not broken down by oral bacteria, such drinks are not cariogenic. However, as the carbonation process means that 'diet' drinks inherently have a very low pH, frequent consumption poses a risk of dental erosion.

Confectionery that uses sugar substitutes as sweetening agents is manufactured and sold using the 'tooth-friendly' logo. Sugar alcohols such as xylitol are used here. However, the side effects of xylitol consumption limit their use, particularly in young children, in whom excess intake can lead to diarrhoea.

The greatest issue yet to be overcome by food scientists is the lack of heat resistance of current sugar substitutes. This limits their use in cooked and baked foods.

Sugar tax

Formally known as the Soft Drinks Industry Levy (SDIL), concerns about obesity led the UK government to implement a two-tiered tax levy on manufacturers of soft drinks in April 2018.

- Drinks ≥8 g sugar/100 mL (high tier) are taxed at £0.24/L
- Drinks ≥5 to <8 g sugar/100 mL (low tier) are taxed at £0.18/L
- Drinks with <5 g sugar/100 mL (no levy) are not taxed.

The SDIL has been widely regarded as a success. It has been estimated that 83% of the reduction in sugar intake seen as a result of the levy can be attributed to a reformulation of high sugar products by manufacturers. The remaining 17% of SDIL-associated reductions in weekly calorie intake from soft drinks were driven by consumers switching towards lower-sugar drinks. By March 2023, it was estimated that the SDIL was responsible for the removal of 45,000 tonnes of sugar from soft drinks in the UK.

Sugar industry

Those involved in the production and marketing of sugar-containing products are resistant to attempts to constrain the sugar market, and the sugar industry has opposed WHO guidelines on the intake of sugars.

The **commercial determinants of health** are now a major focus of public health research. This work aims to develop a better understanding of how commerce harms or benefits health and how regulatory action can be utilised to deliver incentives and investments that advance health, wellbeing and equity in society.

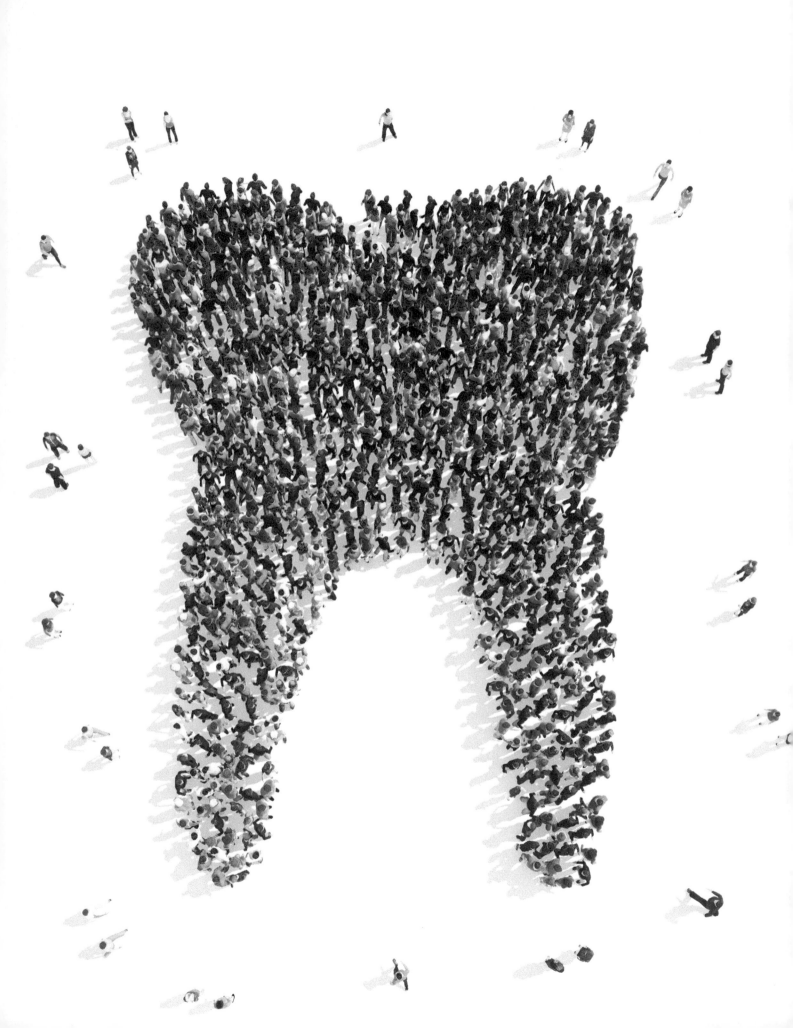

Tobacco and oral health

Part 7

Chapters

31 Tobacco and oral health

Figure 31.1   Global trends in prevalence of tobacco use 2000–2025 (Percentage of population by sex). Source: *Adapted from WHO global report, 2025 (2021).*

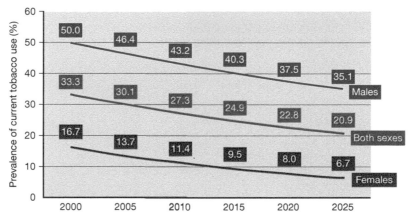

Figure 31.2   Global trends in the number of tobacco users 2000–2025. (By number and sex). Source: *Adapted from WHO global report, 2025 (2021).*

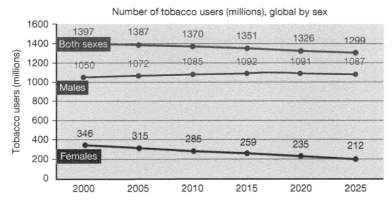

Figure 31.3   Likelihood of smoking compared with base category (England 2016). Source: *Reproduced from Smoking inequalities in England, 2016/Office of National Statistics (2018)/ Crown / Licensed under CC BY 3.0).*

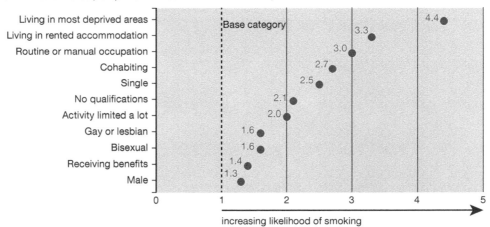

Dental Public Health at a Glance, Second Edition. Ivor G. Chestnutt.
© 2024 John Wiley & Sons Ltd. Published 2024 by John Wiley & Sons Ltd.

Global tobacco use

Tobacco kills more than 8 million people each year. According to the World Health Organisation, more than 7 million of those deaths are the result of direct tobacco use, while around 1.2 million are the result of non-smokers being exposed to second-hand smoke.

The global pattern of tobacco use (smoked and smokeless) is illustrated in Figure 31.1. In the year 2000, one third of the world's population used tobacco (50% males and 16.7% females). If current trends continue, the proportion of the world's population who use tobacco will have reduced to one-fifth by 2025. However, this marked fall in the percentage of the population who smoke is less dramatic when the number of individual tobacco users (mainly smokers) is considered (Figure 31.2). Growth in the world population means that whilst a lesser proportion of the population uses tobacco, the number of users will remain significant, falling from 1397 million in 2000 to 1299 million in 2025. Over 80% of the world's 1.3 billion tobacco users live in low- and middle-income countries. Of the 1326 million tobacco users in 2020, 416 million resided in South East Asian, and 425 million lived in the Western Pacific.

The demographics of tobacco smoking in Great Britain

Trends in tobacco smoking in Great Britain are shown in Figure 32.1 in 1974, just under half the population smoked tobacco. The prevalence of smoking has fallen steadily in the past five decades. In 2021, 15.1% of men (around 3.7 million) and 11.5% of women (around 2.9 million) reported being current smokers.

These average data for the total British population mask an important fact – the association between smoking and social class. Those residents in the most deprived decile of deprivation are 4.4 times more likely to smoke tobacco than those living in the least deprived decile (Figure 31.3). Smoking is a major contributor to inequalities in health. The likelihood of increased smoking, associated with other demographic characteristics, is also shown in Figure 31.3.

Smoking varies across ethnic groups, with marked differences between the proportion of men and the proportion of women who smoke in some ethnicities (Table 31.1).

Tobacco and general health

Tobacco consumption is recognised as the United Kingdom's single greatest cause of preventable illness and early death. About 78,000 individuals in the UK die as a result of smoking every year, and many more have a reduced quality of life or live with a debilitating disease as a result of smoking tobacco. Smoking is known to increase the risk of developing more than 50 serious health conditions. The effects of smoking are not confined to those who smoke. Passive smoking (breathing tobacco smoke produced by others) can be lethal to non-smokers.

Passive smoking

Non-smokers who live with a smoking partner or who work in an environment where levels of tobacco smoke are high, such as pubs and bars, are at increased risk of developing a smoking-related disease. Recognition of the impact of second-hand tobacco smoke has been instrumental in the introduction of legislation prohibiting smoking in public places. Smoking during pregnancy is likely to have an adverse impact on the health of the foetus.

Tobacco and oral health

Tobacco, whether smoked or used in a smokeless form, has impacts on oral health in many ways (Table 31.2).

Table 31.1 Percentage of adults in the UK who currently smoke cigarettes by ethnicity and sex, 2021

Ethnicity	Percentage of adults	
	Male	Female
Asian	13.0	2.6
Black	9.0	7.2
Chinese	9.4	1.9
Mixed	18.6	12.9
White	15.3	12.4
Other	15.4	6.2

Source: *Office for National Statistics: Smoking habits in the UK and its constituent countries 2021.*

Table 31.2 The effect of tobacco use on oral health

Condition	Observations
Hairy tongue	Caused by increased keratinisation of the filiform papillae this is a benign condition that is most commonly seen in smokers. It may assume a brown or black colour due to the presence of chromogenic bacteria.
Halitosis	Probably the most common effect of smoking – can be used as a motivator to encourage young people to quit smoking.
Keratosis	Thickening of the oral mucosa, particularly in areas directly exposed to the thermal trauma of cigarette smoke, results in a white appearance and increased keratin layer on the mucosal surface. Nicotinic stomatitis affecting the palate and buccal mucosa are commonly affected sites.
Leukoplakia	White patches, which may be precancerous, are more commonly seen in smokers.
Oral cancer	The most serious effect of tobacco use on the oral cavity is that smoking cigarettes increases the risk of oral cancer 2–4 times. Smoking has a synergistic effect when combined with heavy alcohol consumption, which together increase the risk of developing oral cancer 6–15 times.
Periodontal disease	Smoking cigarettes will increase the risk of periodontal attachment loss by 2–5 times. However, periodontal disease in smokers can be masked by the vasoconstrictive effects of nicotine on the gingival tissues, resulting in a lack of bleeding and the obvious redness pathognomonic of gingivitis.
Sinusitis	The irritant effects of cigarette smoke predisposes to sinusitis.
Tooth staining	Smoking, often in combination with poor oral hygiene, is a common cause of external tooth discolouration. Staining can be used as a motivating factor to help discuss smoking cessation in a non-threatening way with patients.
Wound healing	Smokers frequently have an impaired ability to heal – alveolar osteitis (dry socket) is seen more commonly in smokers. Patients who smoke respond less well to both non-surgical and surgical periodontal therapy.

32 Alternative ways in which tobacco is used and tobacco control

Figure 32.1 The proportion of the population in Great Britain who smoked cigarettes from 1974 to 2019 and tobacco control legislative interventions

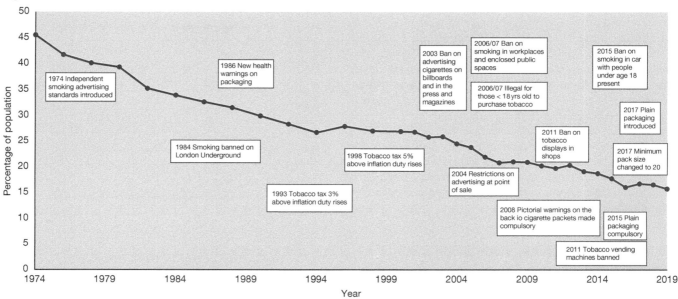

Table 32.1 Summary of the effects of using a waterpipe to smoke tobacco

Using a waterpipe to smoke tobacco poses a serious potential health hazard to smokers and others exposed to the smoke emitted.

Using a waterpipe to smoke tobacco is not a safe alternative to cigarette smoking.

A typical one-hour-long waterpipe smoking session involves inhaling 100–200 times the volume of smoke inhaled with a single cigarette.

Even after it has been passed through water, the smoke produced by a waterpipe contains high levels of toxic compounds, including carbon monoxide, heavy metals and cancer-causing chemicals.

Commonly used heat sources that are applied to burn tobacco, such as wood cinders or charcoal, are likely to increase the health risks because when such fuels are combusted, they produce their own toxicants, including high levels of carbon monoxide, metals and cancer-causing chemicals.

Pregnant women and the foetus are particularly vulnerable when exposed either actively or involuntarily to the waterpipe smoke and toxicants.

Second-hand smoke from waterpipes is a mixture of tobacco smoke in addition to the smoke from the fuel and, therefore, poses a serious risk for non-smokers.

There is no proof that any device or accessory can make waterpipe smoking safer.

Sharing a waterpipe mouthpiece poses a serious risk of transmission of communicable diseases, including tuberculosis and hepatitis.

Waterpipe tobacco is often sweetened and flavoured, making it very appealing; the sweet smell and taste of the smoke may explain why some people, particularly young people who otherwise would not use tobacco, begin to use waterpipes.

Source: *WHO (2015a).*

Table 32.2 E-cigarettes – Vaping – Current evidence

Use

In 2022, 8.6% of young people (aged 11–18) vaped, either occasionally or regularly, up from 4.8% in 2020

7.0% of adults in England reported vaping in 2021.

In 2021 vaping prevalence among adults who have never smoked was estimated as between 0.6% and 0.7%.

Most young people who have never smoked are also not currently vaping (98.3%)

Risks

In the short and medium term, vaping poses a small fraction of the risks of smoking.

Studies assessing longer-term risk are required.

Vaping is not risk-free, particularly for people who have never smoked.

Flavours

Fruit flavours remained the most popular among adults and young people who vape, followed by 'menthol/mint'.

Overall, there is a lack of evidence on whether flavourings affect health risks.

Aid to stopping smoking

Vaping products remain the most common aid used by people to help them stop smoking.

In stop-smoking services from 2020 to 2021, quit attempts involving a vaping product were associated with the highest success rates (64.9% compared with 58.6% for attempts not involving a vaping product)

Source: *Adapted from Office for Health Improvement and Disparities (2022).*

Alternative ways in which tobacco is used

Tobacco is most commonly smoked in the form of cigarettes, either manufactured or as 'roll-ups'. Smoking cigars or a pipe is a less frequent form of consumption. However, it is common in many ethnic groups for tobacco to be used in other ways, all of which are prejudicial to oral health.

Bidis

Bidis are small, hand-rolled cigarettes typically smoked in India and other South East Asian countries. They produce three times more carbon monoxide and five times more tar than regular cigarettes.

Shisha, hookas, waterpipes

Shisha, tobacco cured with flavourings and smoked from waterpipes (also known as hookas or hubble-bubbles), is used by an estimated 100 million people worldwide. Originating in Middle Eastern countries, it is becoming increasingly common in Europe and North America. The moistened tobacco is placed in a bowl over hot coals, and the smoke is drawn by a pipe through water. The use of tobacco in this format poses risks to general and oral health (Table 32.1).

Betel quid

Betel quid is a combination of betel leaf, areca nut and slaked lime. With or without tobacco, it is widely used in Asia and the Pacific region. It is also used by people resident in the United Kingdom whose origins are in Asia. Placed in the buccal sulcus, the quid has a mildly stimulant effect. Use predisposes to the development of precancerous conditions: leukoplakia, erythroplakia and oral submucous fibrosis (OSF). OSF is common in the Indian subcontinent and presents as a thickening of the oral soft tissues, which limits the opening of the mouth.

Gutkha

Gutkha is a smokeless tobacco mixture that is sweetened and spiced. It is sold in foil packets, and the highly coloured packaging makes it attractive to children and young people.

Tobacco and recreational drugs

Cannabis (marijuana) is commonly smoked in combination with tobacco. Smokers of 'weed' commonly present with the intraoral signs common in those who smoke conventional cigarettes.

Dipping tobacco (moist snuff)

This mode of tobacco use originates in Scandinavia. A bolus of tobacco is placed in the buccal sulcus, and the nicotine is absorbed via the oral tissues. It is sold either loose in tins or in bags resembling tea bags. Its use predisposes the individual to oral cancer. Made popular by American baseball stars, dipping tobacco still poses a problem among US teenagers.

E-cigarettes and vaping

E-cigarettes do not contain tobacco. They produce an aerosol by heating a liquid that may or may not contain nicotine. The aerosol is inhaled to provide the sensation of inhaling tobacco smoke without the smoke – 'vaping' is the term that describes the use of the devices. The solution contains various flavours. There has been a significant debate on the merits of vaping devices as an aid to stopping smoking. The Office of Health Improvement and Disparities is of the view that emerging evidence confirms that e-cigarettes have an important role to play in harm reduction as an alternative to smoking tobacco and aid to stopping smoking (Table 32.2). However, significant concerns are emerging about the use of vaping devices by schoolchildren, especially a worry that they may prove a pathway to smoking tobacco.

Approaches to tobacco control

Approaches to controlling tobacco can be divided into:
- Control measures aimed at a population level (upstream).
- Control measures aimed at helping individuals stop smoking (downstream).

Population-level tobacco control measures

Health departments in the United Kingdom have introduced a range of tobacco control measures (Figure 32.1). The ban on smoking in enclosed work and public spaces is one of the most significant public health measures to have been implemented in recent decades.

Bans on tobacco advertising, promotion and sponsorship can reduce tobacco consumption. Tobacco taxes are one of the most cost-effective ways of reducing tobacco use, especially among young people and the poor. The World Health Organization suggests that a tax increase that raises the price of tobacco by 10% decreases tobacco consumption by about 4% in high-income countries and by up to 8% in low- and middle-income countries. Taxation has, over the years, been a key weapon against tobacco use in the United Kingdom. However, this means of control is undermined by the ready availability of smuggled contraband and fake tobacco brands on the black market. Tobacco smuggling undermines efforts to reduce smoking prevalence and costs the UK taxpayer an estimated £2.2 billion per annum.

Stopping smoking

Given the impact of tobacco on health, stopping people from taking up smoking or helping them cease the habit if they already use tobacco is one of the great challenges facing public health. One-half of all smokers will die directly as a result of their habit. In surveys, around 7 in 10 smokers report that they would like to give up smoking, and just under 4 in 10 smokers have tried to do so in the past 12 months. Five out of six smokers claim that they would not start smoking had they had the choice to make it again.

Nicotine, a psychoactive substance that acts on receptors in the brain, is highly addictive. Overcoming dependence on nicotine is a key element in giving up smoking. Nicotine withdrawal symptoms can include irritability, anxiety, difficulty concentrating and increased appetite. Stopping smoking is difficult, and those who successfully quit often report several failed attempts before finally kicking the habit.

The benefits of stopping smoking

Smoking cessation:
- Lowers the risk of lung and other types of cancer
- Reduces the risk of coronary heart disease, stroke and peripheral vascular disease. Coronary heart disease risk is substantially reduced within one to two years of quitting
- Reduces respiratory symptoms such as coughing, wheezing and shortness of breath and also reduces the risk of developing chronic obstructive pulmonary disease
- Reduces staining of the teeth and halitosis
- Increases the chances of a successful outcome following the placement of dental implants or periodontal surgery.

As described in Chapter 33, members of the dental team have an important role to play in helping smokers give up.

33 Smoking cessation

Figure 33.1 The stages of change model applied to smoking cessation in a dental setting. Source: *Adapted from Prochaska and DiClemente (1982).*

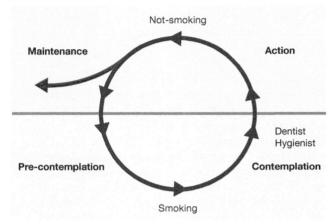

Figure 33.2 Very brief advice on smoking

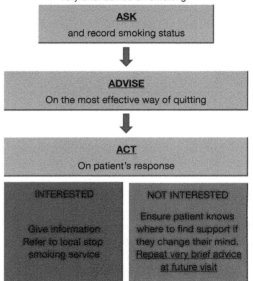

Table 33.1 The effectiveness of interventions in helping smokers to stop smoking

Interventions (in order of decreasing effectiveness)	Effectiveness
Local stop smoking services	Offer the best chance of success. These centres have specially trained counsellors who can combine smoking aids (nicotine replacement/medication) with expert behavioural support. Smokers wishing to quit are **three times** as likely to be successful if they attend a stop smoking service than if they go it alone using willpower only.
Stop smoking medication prescribed by a medical practitioner or pharmacist, or other health professional	Medicines will **double** the chances of quitting compared with willpower alone.
Over-the-counter nicotine replacement such as patches, gum or e-cigarettes	Nicotine replacement therapy will increase the changes of quitting by **one and a half times** compared to will-power
Will-power alone	The least effective method (although many people have stopped smoking using this method).
Acupuncture	A 2014 Cochrane systematic review found no evidence that acupuncture or associated acupressure was helpful in assisting smokers to quit, but noted that a lack of consistent evidence meant that no firm conclusions could be drawn. Although safe when correctly applied, acupuncture is likely to be less effective than current evidence-based interventions in helping smokers give up.
Hypnotherapy	A 2019 Cochrane systematic review concluded that there is insufficient evidence to determine whether hypnotherapy is more effective for smoking cessation than other forms of behavioural support or unassisted quitting.

Dental Public Health at a Glance, Second Edition. Ivor G. Chestnutt.
© 2024 John Wiley & Sons Ltd. Published 2024 by John Wiley & Sons Ltd.

Individual smoking cessation – the process of stopping smoking

A number of behaviour change theories have been applied to help individuals stop smoking. One of the most popular is the Stages of Change or Trans-theoretical Model of Change proposed by American psychologists Prochasksa and DiClemente. This model suggests that people move through a series of motivational stages before they succeed in stopping smoking (Figure 33.1). The majority of smokers are at any one time in a **pre-contemplation stage** (not thinking about quitting). A minority of smokers are at any one time thinking about giving up – the **contemplation stage**. Some will then take action and stop smoking – the **action stage**. Some manage to stay stopped and enter the **maintenance stage** (stopped smoking for more than six months). However, many will fail and relapse before going on to try a further quit attempt.

While some smokers manage to stay stopped after the first attempt, many will go around the quit and relapse circle a number of times before finally managing to stay stopped. In some ways, the process can be viewed as learning and practising. Many smoking-cessation programmes aim to identify the stage that a smoker is in at a given time and attempt to tailor cessation information appropriately.

A Cochrane review of stage-based interventions for smoking cessation concluded that approaches based on stages of change were neither more nor less effective than interventions that were not based on such an approach.

What helps smokers to quit?

There is no good evidence on what is effective in helping smokers stop smoking. The effectiveness of different interventions is summarised in Table 33.1. The most effective method is a combination of behavioural support and stop-smoking medication.

Behavioural support/advice and counselling

Brief advice from a healthcare professional will increase the chances of stopping smoking, but success with quitting increases with multiple sessions – usually six weekly sessions with a trained counsellor. Counselling can be conducted in person, individually or in groups, or via telephone helplines. Interactive websites also provide helpful information and assistance to those who are attempting to stop smoking.

Medication

Continuance of smoking is heavily influenced by dependence on nicotine. The provision of nicotine-replacement therapy (NRT) significantly increases the chances of a successful quit attempt. NRT is available in a range of delivery vehicles: chewing gum, skin patches, lozenges and nasal spray. There is evidence that e-cigarettes can be effective in helping smokers stop smoking, albeit the long-term effects of using e-cigarettes await determination (Table 32.2).

There are drugs available on prescription (but not by dentists) that are effective in helping smokers stop smoking.

Varenicline (Champix) prevents nicotine from reaching nicotine receptors in the brain and also stimulates dopamine production, both of which make cigarette smoking less satisfying.

Bupropion (Zyban) works by blocking nicotinic receptors and thus reduces the craving for nicotine. A side effect of this medication, which was originally used as an antidepressant, is dryness of the mouth.

Smoking cessation services

Across the United Kingdom, a range of smoking-cessation services have been established to help smokers give up. These services employ trained counsellors who have the skills to deliver both behavioural support and facilitate access to medicines and nicotine replacement therapy. They provide interactive websites and telephone helplines. Dental patients who express an interest in quitting should be referred directly to their local stop-smoking service.

The role of the dental team in providing smoking-cessation advice

Members of the dental team are in an ideal position to identify patients who smoke and who are contemplating giving up. Dentists are often the only healthcare professionals who see healthy young adults who are smokers on a regular basis. Smoking status should form a core question in taking a patient's medical history. This can act as a prompt to 'very brief advice on smoking'. There are three steps in this process: Ask, Advise and Act, as illustrated in Figure 33.2. It is suggested that this process take about 30 seconds.

Having identified patients who are interested in stopping smoking, dentists should refer them to the local smoking-cessation services, which have the expertise to provide appropriate counselling and can prescribe effective medication to help overcome nicotine withdrawal. Those not interested in stopping should be asked again at a future visit to check if they have changed their mind. Given the cyclical nature of smoking-cessation attempts, it is useful to enquire about progress at subsequent appointments, even for those who have engaged.

The dental team can be disheartened by apparently only seeing a small number of those approached to take up the offer of help and quit. However, the public health benefits come not from the success rate of an individual practitioner or practice but from the collective efforts of the profession. Even if each dental professional only sees one or two patients quit per year, the contribution to public health and lives saved from the collective effort of every dentist, hygienist, therapist or oral health educator in the country is enormous.

Remember, for each patient that stops smoking after one year, their chances of a heart attack will have halved compared with a smoker's. After 10 years, the risk of death from lung cancer will have halved compared with having continued to smoke!

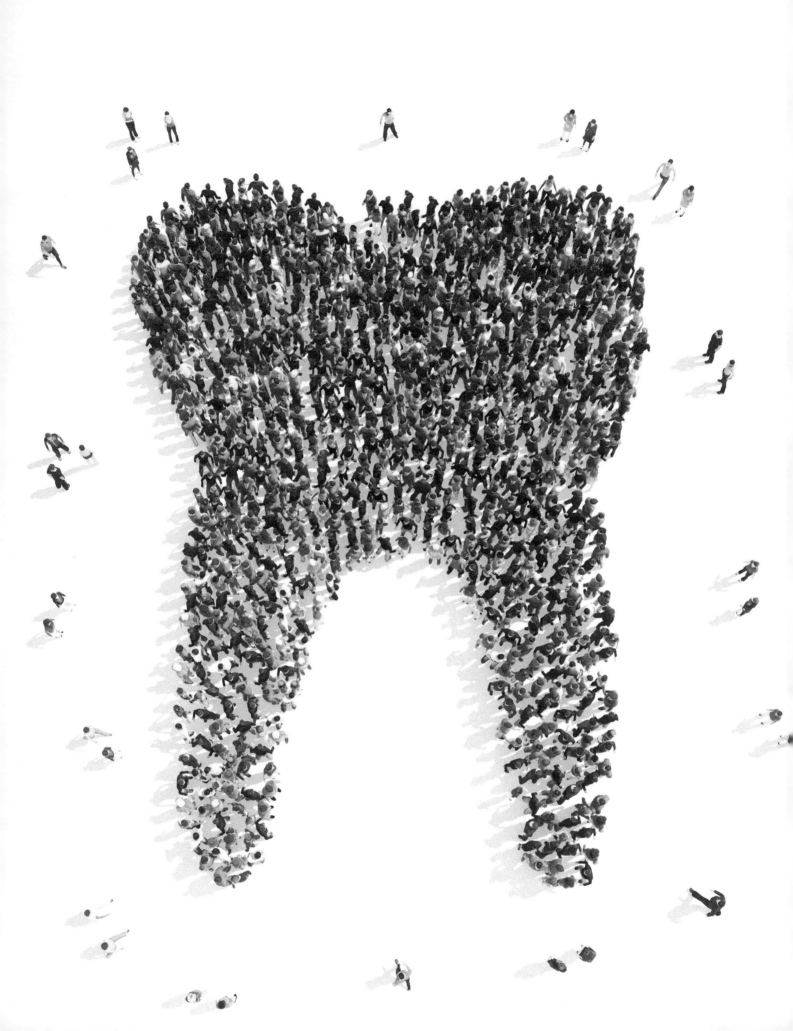

Alcohol and oral health

34 Alcohol and oral health

Figure 34.1 Impact of alcohol on oral health and dentistry

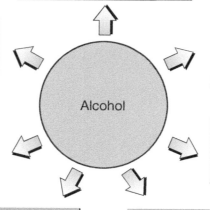

Alcohol is a risk factor for oral cancer

Management of patients with alcohol induced health problems, e.g. reduced clotting times

Trauma to oral and facial tissues can occur when patients are drunk

Dental professionals themselves may be at risk from excess use of alcohol

Alcohol

Consumption of excess alcoholic drinks of low pH (e.g. wine) can result in non-carious tooth surface loss - as can gastric reflux associated with alcohol abuse

Dentists and their team may, by providing brief advice, make patients aware of their alcohol consumption

Dental professionals can identify people with potentially harmful patterns of alcohol consumption when taking a medical history

Table 34.1 Advice on minimising risk from drinking alcohol.

Weekly Drinking Guide

This applies to adults who drink regularly or frequently, i.e. most weeks

The Chief Medical Officers' guideline for both men and women is that:
• To keep health risks from alcohol to a low level, it is safest not to drink more than 14 units a week on a regular basis.
• If you regularly drink as much as 14 units per week, it is best to spread your drinking evenly over three or more days. If you have one or two heavy drinking episodes a week, you increase your risks of death from long-term illness and from accidents and injuries.
• The risk of developing a range of health problems (including cancers of the mouth, throat and breast) increases the more you drink on a regular basis.
• If you wish to cut down the amount you drink, a good way to help achieve this is to have several drink-free days each week.

Single Occasion Drinking Episodes

This applies to drinking on any single occasion (not regular drinking, which is covered by the weekly guideline)

The Chief Medical Officers' advice for men and women who wish to keep their short-term health risks from single-occasion drinking episodes to a low level is to reduce them by:
• limiting the total amount of alcohol you drink on any single occasion.
• drinking more slowly, drinking with food, and alternating with water.
• planning ahead to avoid problems, e.g. by making sure you can get home safely or that you have people you trust with you.

Pregnancy and Drinking

This applies to those who are pregnant or are trying to become pregnant

The Chief Medical Officers' guideline is that:
• If you are pregnant or think you could become pregnant, the safest approach is not to drink alcohol at all to keep risks to your baby to a minimum.
• Drinking in pregnancy can lead to long-term harm to the baby, with the more you drink, the greater the risk.

Source: *Adapted from UK Chief Medical Officers' Low Risk Drinking Guidelines.*

Table 34.2 Definition of a unit of alcohol and examples of units contained in typical drinks

Definition of a unit of alcohol	1 unit = 10 ml by volume or 8 g by weight of pure alcohol
Examples	
1 unit of alcohol	One-half pint of ordinary-strength beer, lager or cider (3–4% ABV)
1 unit of alcohol	A small pub measure of spirits – 25 ml (40% ABV)
1.5 units of alcohol	Small glass (125 ml) wine (ABV 12%)
3 units of alcohol	One-half litre (500 ml, just under a pint) of strong beer (6% ABV)
3.5 units of alcohol	Large glass (250 ml) wine (ABV 14%)

Alcohol and health

The consumption of alcohol is an integral part of the social fabric of most developed and many developing countries. While alcohol is a legal commodity, consumption of alcohol is associated with risk. The Chief Medical Officers in the United Kingdom have issued guidance to enable people to make informed choices about their alcohol intake (Tables 34.1 and 34.2). The guidance covers three areas: advice to those who drink most weeks, advice about consuming alcohol on any single occasion and guidance for those who are pregnant or are considering becoming pregnant.

In the UK, there are currently over 10 million people drinking at levels that increase their risk of health harm. While the average age of death from all causes in England is 77.6 years, the average age of those dying from an alcohol-specific cause is 54.3 years. Annually, 1 million hospital admissions can be broadly related to alcohol and alcohol accounts for 10% of the burden of disease and death. The government estimates that alcohol-related harm currently costs the National Health Service £3.7 billion every year (equal to £120 for every taxpayer) and wider UK society more than £21 billion – more than double the £10 billion revenue generated from alcohol taxes.

Surveys show that a large proportion of the population routinely exceeds the recommended limits. Excess consumption occurs in two main ways: long-term regular (daily) exposure to alcohol and binge drinking, where the safe levels of consumption are regularly exceeded, interspersed with periods of no or limited drinking. The latter pattern of consumption has been particularly common in young people in the United Kingdom in recent years. Some people's consumption of alcohol reaches a stage where they become addicted and on a journey that often results in them losing everything in their life and eventually life itself; they are termed alcoholics. The common diseases related to excess alcohol consumption are shown in Table 34.3.

In addition to the impact on health, alcohol-related crime, disorder and domestic violence are significant social consequences of alcohol misuse.

Alcohol and dentistry

Alcohol can have impacts on dentistry and oral health in a number of ways (Figure 34.1). It is a well-recognised risk factor for oral cancer, particularly in combination with smoking tobacco. Alcohol can also affect treatment, either by causing oral-facial trauma, by leading to systemic disease (e.g. liver disease) that complicates patient management, or when patients present for treatment under the influence of alcohol. Alcohol-reduction advice by dental professionals will be discussed shortly.

Dentistry is recognised as a potentially stressful occupation, and recourse to alcohol use in excess is an occupational hazard. Members of the dental team have a duty to be aware of their own alcohol consumption and to watch out for signs of alcohol abuse in colleagues and employees.

Actions to reduce alcohol misuse

At a population level

Upstream actions to reduce alcohol misuse vary from country to country. For instance, in Scandinavia, the sale of alcohol is very strictly controlled, and it can only be purchased from special points of sale. In other countries, alcohol is readily available, too readily available in the view of many healthcare professionals. While legislation exists to prohibit the sale of alcohol to minors, there is great concern at the ease with which this can be circumvented, enabling teenagers and adolescents to access alcohol.

Minimum Unit Pricing (MUP), set at 50 pence per unit, has been introduced in Scotland (2018) and Wales (2020) but not to date in England. Advocates for public health suggest that this will curb the sale of cheap high-strength alcoholic drinks by supermarkets and corner shops – often suspected as the sources of alcohol purchased by or on behalf of minors. Opponents have argued that rather than legislate for a minimum alcohol unit price; it is preferable to work with the drinks industry to achieve agreement on the pricing and marketing of alcohol, particularly to young people and adolescents, by responsible advertising and drinks promotions. MUP is supported by the World Health Organisation. The full impact of MUP's effectiveness as an alcohol control measure awaits determination, but there is emerging evidence of a reduction of alcohol-attributable harm in Scotland.

The debate on MUP for alcohol is a good illustration of the concept of the '**nanny state**'. A perennial problem for public health is to what extent the government should legislate to influence and control people's lifestyles and life circumstances or whether this should be left to market and other forces to decide. Obviously, a sensible balance needs to be struck between over-regulation for health and a free-for-all, where people fail to act in their own best interests or in those of fellow members of society.

At an individual level

It has also been suggested that as part of their overall holistic care of patients, members of the dental team are in a good position to identify those who are consuming more than the safe level of alcohol. The argument is that dentists, therapists and hygienists see fit and healthy patients who may not otherwise have routine contact with a healthcare professional. While dentist involvement in alcohol-related advice has been explored in the context of drunk patients attending Accident and Emergency departments with facial injuries, the potential for dentists to get involved in alcohol-reduction advice in dental practice has yet to be fully investigated. It certainly has not been considered to the same extent as dentists' involvement in smoking cessation advice.

Screening questions on a medical history form may highlight a patient with excess alcohol consumption. The Fast Alcohol Screening Test (FAST) is a way of identifying those whose alcohol intake is a cause for concern. Giving brief motivational advice and 'maximising the teachable moment' is held as important action to help patients moderate their alcohol intake. An example is when a patient who has been involved in an alcohol-inspired fight requires stitches for facial trauma. When they return to have their wound checked, are sober, and have had the chance to reflect on the events that led to their injury, they may be susceptible to brief alcohol-reduction advice.

The key current issues in this regard are the degree to which dental practitioners feel prepared to ask patients about their drinking and whether they are properly equipped to advise patients identified as in need of alcohol-reduction advice and to make the necessary onward referral to the patient's general medical practitioner. In addition, patients' expectations of being asked about their drinking when attending a dental professional may be a further issue.

Table 34.3 Health complications of excess alcohol consumption

Health complications of excess alcohol consumption
Liver disease (cirrhosis or hepatitis)
Cancer
Gut and pancreas disorders
Depression
Anxiety
Sexual difficulties
Hypertension
Accidents/trauma
Obesity

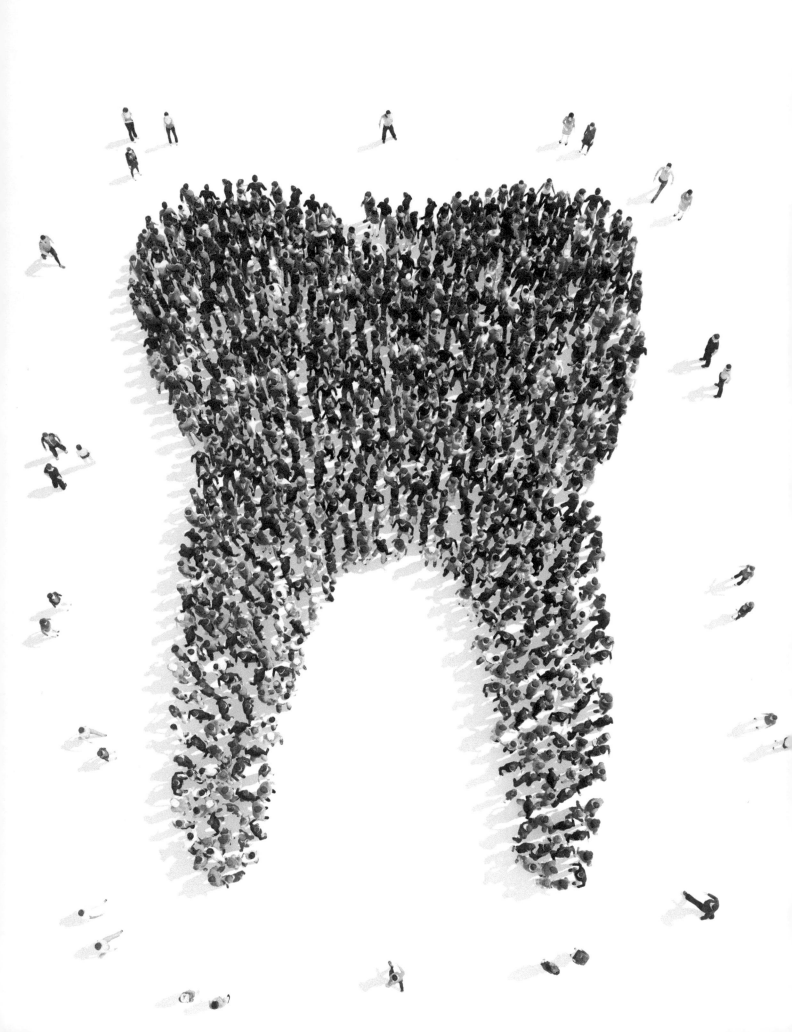

Assessing health needs

Part 9

Chapters

Assessing oral health needs on a population basis

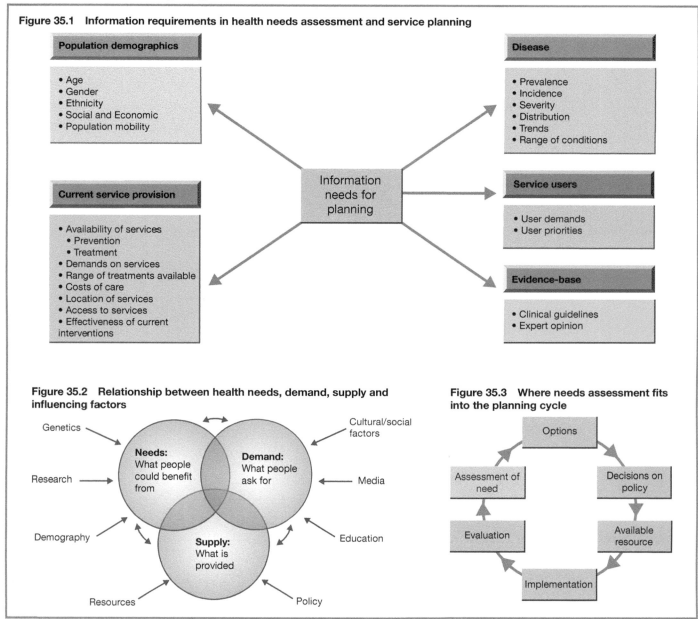

Figure 35.1 Information requirements in health needs assessment and service planning

Population demographics
- Age
- Gender
- Ethnicity
- Social and Economic
- Population mobility

Current service provision
- Availability of services
  - Prevention
  - Treatment
- Demands on services
- Range of treatments available
- Costs of care
- Location of services
- Access to services
- Effectiveness of current interventions

Information needs for planning

Disease
- Prevalence
- Incidence
- Severity
- Distribution
- Trends
- Range of conditions

Service users
- User demands
- User priorities

Evidence-base
- Clinical guidelines
- Expert opinion

Figure 35.2 Relationship between health needs, demand, supply and influencing factors

Genetics

Research

Demography

Resources

Needs: What people could benefit from

Demand: What people ask for

Supply: What is provided

Cultural/social factors

Media

Education

Policy

Figure 35.3 Where needs assessment fits into the planning cycle

Options

Decisions on policy

Available resource

Implementation

Evaluation

Assessment of need

Determining oral health needs

For an individual patient

When treating a patient in a clinical setting, a dentist will gather facts about the individual by asking questions and undertaking a clinical examination. The information gathered, possibly supplemented by special tests or investigations, will enable the dentist to diagnose the patient's condition. In consultation with the patient, the dentist will be able to assess the patient's needs and discuss treatment options, from which a treatment plan can be formulated and agreed. This process is known as **diagnosis and treatment planning**.

For a population

In dental public health, a similar process occurs, although instead of considering the needs of an individual patient, a public health dentist has to consider the needs of a population or subgroup within a population. This process is known as **oral health needs assessment**.

Oral health needs assessment

Oral health needs assessment involves:
- Examining and describing the characteristics of the population
- Identifying their needs, including the wishes of the population

Dental Public Health at a Glance, Second Edition. Ivor G. Chestnutt.
© 2024 John Wiley & Sons Ltd. Published 2024 by John Wiley & Sons Ltd.

- Examining current service provision and its capacity to meet the needs of the population
- Where gaps exist, identify how these can be met, either by reorganising existing services, investing in new services or decommissioning services that are no longer required or fit for purpose.

The purpose of oral health needs assessment is to:
- Identify and quantify oral health needs
- Identify potential health gains
- Permit prioritisation of identified needs
- Inform the planning and commissioning of oral health services.

An understanding of how to assess oral health needs is, therefore, a fundamental component of dental public health practice.

How to conduct an oral health needs assessment

Needs can be viewed from different perspectives, such as normative/expressed/felt/comparative needs, as discussed in Chapter 42.

Needs assessment can also be conducted from a range of perspectives:

Epidemiological
- Disease prevalence/incidence in distinct geographical localities, e.g. caries prevalence in different local authority areas
- Specific diseases, e.g. oral cancer incidence in older men from disadvantaged backgrounds.

Comparative
- Comparing services/providers in different localities, e.g. waiting lists for orthodontic treatment.

Corporate
- Draws on the views of different groups, e.g. providers of healthcare on the provision of oral care for nursing home residents and local people on the provision of out-of-hours dental care.

Information used in health needs planning is shown in Figure 35.1.

Need, demand and supply

In addition to **need**, there are two other factors that have to be considered when planning and delivering a health service. These are **demand** and **supply**.

Need is what people could benefit from, for instance, greater provision of NHS dentistry in a given area.

Demand is what people want, such as easier access to NHS dentistry, expressed perhaps by letters of complaint to local public representatives.

Supply is what is provided, for example, the existing number of dentists accepting patients for NHS care.

The relationship between health needs, demand and supply and the factors that influence them are shown in Figure 35.2.

The planning cycle

Health service planning should ideally be a cyclical process, where needs assessment forms a vital role in informing the options available. However, the process of planning is often constrained by the resources available and by political influences on health service provision. The place of health needs assessment in the planning cycle is shown in Figure 35.3.

The role of local authorities in service planning

England

Joint local health and wellbeing strategies
Local Authorities have statutory powers over service areas including planning, housing, benefits, and leisure and green spaces, which affect many of the most significant determinants of health. The Health and Social Care Act 2012 in England transferred much of the responsibility for public health from the National Health Service to local authorities. This has been further modified by the Health and Care Act of 2022, which established **integrated care boards (ICBs)** and **integrated care partnerships (ICPs)** (Chapter 39).

Planning in local authorities is undertaken by **Health and Wellbeing Boards (HWBs)**. Their decision-making is guided by a **joint strategic needs assessment (JSNA)**. This is defined as a process that identifies current and future health and wellbeing needs in the light of existing services and informs future service planning, taking into account evidence of effectiveness. A JSNA identifies the 'big picture', in terms of the health and wellbeing needs and inequalities of a local population. Producing a JSNA is a mandatory requirement designed to help organisations with service planning and the commissioning process. From the JSNA, a **Joint Health and Wellbeing Strategy (JHWS)** is produced with the intention of improving the health and wellbeing results of the local community and reducing inequalities for all ages.

Health and Wellbeing Boards
Health and Wellbeing Boards (HWBs) are designed as a forum where health and social care work together to improve the health and wellbeing of their local population and reduce health inequalities. Each top-tier and unitary authority has its own HWB. The membership of HWBs is mandated in law and includes a local elected representative (councillor), senior staff from the local authority and integrated care boards and the Director of Public Health.

Wales
In Wales, Health Boards and local government have a joint statutory duty to develop a Health, Social Care and Wellbeing Strategy. This focuses on:
- Improving health and wellbeing and reducing inequalities
- The provision, quality, integration and sustainability of services that are provided jointly by health and social services, e.g. nursing, care and residential homes.

Scotland
The way in which health and social care services are planned and delivered in Scotland is governed by the Public Bodies (Joint Working) (Scotland) Act 2014. Local authorities and health boards are required by law to work together to plan and deliver adult community health and social care services. In total, 31 health and social care partnerships have been set up across Scotland.

36 The oral health needs of specific population groups

Box 36.1 Special care dentistry

Special Care Dentistry (SCD)
Special Care Dentistry (SCD) is recognised as a distinct dental specialty. Dentists with appropriate postgraduate training and experience can apply to the General Dental Council (GDC) for entry to the Specialist List in SCD. The GDC describes SCD as 'providing preventive and treatment oral care services for adults who are unable to accept routine dental care because of some physical, intellectual, medical, emotional, sensory, mental or social impairment, or a combination of these factors'.

Box 36.2 Prison dentistry

Prison Dentistry
Providing dental care for prisoners poses a number of challenges.
  Issues include:
• Prisoners' oral health is among the poorest in any group. The majority of prisoners come from areas of low social and economic status, and their oral health is said to be four times worse than that of their peers.
• Prisoners have significant general health issues that can complicate their dental management. These include poor mental health, illegal drug use, and dependency on alcohol and tobacco.
• Prior to imprisonment many prisoners were sporadic dental attenders, many attending only when in pain.
• Implementing oral hygiene regimes in prison needs to account for potential security issues to prevent oral hygiene aids from being used as weapons.
• Most prisons have in-house dental surgery, but the efficiency of dental services can be low, with only a few prisoners being seen in each treatment session. This can be attributed to the need for prisoners to be escorted to the prison for dental surgery, and patients may refuse to attend at the last minute.
• A 2018 survey has shown that equipment and facilities in many prisons need replacing or upgrading.
• Many prisoners are anxious about dental treatment, having had limited exposure to dental care prior to incarceration.
• The transient nature of the prison population: prisoners move from remand to longer-term prisons; prisoners are moved from one institution to another; and the short sentences that many prisoners serve mean that completing a course of treatment can be problematic.

Box 36.3 Armed forces dentistry

Armed Forces Dentistry
The military forms a distinct group within the population whose dental care needs require special consideration.

In the United Kingdom, dental care for soldiers, sailors, airmen and their families is provided by the Defence Dental Service (DDS). The DDS is a tri-service organization employing personnel from the Royal Navy, Army, Royal Air Force and civilian sector who are trained dentists, hygienists, technicians or dental nurses, as well as critical support staff. Most treatment is provided at service establishments (dental centres) in the United Kingdom and in centres where the British military is permanently deployed. Military dentists are appointed as officers and undergo 14 weeks of basic military training before their first posting. A limited number of cadetships are available to dental students in the United Kingdom.

There are a number of specific issues in providing care for military personnel:
• A high level of oral fitness needs to be secured for military personnel before they are deployed on operational tours of duty. Oral health is viewed as an important element of overall medical fitness for duty.
• Two groups of military personnel require especially good attention to oral health:
  • Submariners – who may be at sea for months at a time.
  • Jet pilots – the high gravitational forces experienced while flying lead to barometric changes that can result in toothache in moribund pulp chambers and around leaking restorations.
• Many of the young men and women recruited to the infantry come from low social and economic circumstances and may have higher disease experience as a result. They require an intensive course of dental treatment to make them dentally fit and thus fit for service.

Dental Public Health at a Glance, Second Edition. Ivor G. Chestnutt.
© 2024 John Wiley & Sons Ltd. Published 2024 by John Wiley & Sons Ltd.

In society, there are groups who share common characteristics that require particular consideration in the commissioning and organisation of their dental care.

People with physical and mental disabilities

Many people with physical and mental disabilities will be able to undergo routine dental care in the General Dental Service. However, those whose disabilities are more severe may require care from a clinician experienced in the provision of special/additional care (Box 36.1). Such patients are frequently cared for by the Community (Salaried/Public) Dental Service. For those patients who require care using general anaesthesia, admission to the Hospital Dental Service may be required. The British Society for Disability and Oral Health has issued guidelines for caring for those with physical and mental disabilities.

Issues include:
- Prevention – providing appropriately tailored primary prevention
- Physical access to surgeries (for wheelchairs/steps/stairs)
- The availability of specialised equipment, e.g. hoists to lift patients into the dental chair, equipment that can recline the patient's own wheelchair, a bariatric chair (to accommodate patients whose body weight exceeds the capacity of a conventional dental chair)
- Access to general anaesthetic/conscious sedation services
- Knowledge of and compliance with the requirements of the Mental Capacity Act 2005 to ensure valid consent
- Making certain that patients are managed in a holistic fashion, to ensure that their dental care is integrated into other complex needs.

Frail elderly people

The increased number of older people, the majority of whom will increasingly have their own teeth (Chapter 9), merits consideration as a specific population group, particularly the frail elderly. These people are often residents in care homes and depend on others for many, if not all, aspects of daily living.

Issues include:
- As more old people retain their own teeth, the need to ensure adequate oral hygiene will assume increasing importance. This will necessitate education for carers on how to provide this.
- An individual oral health needs assessment should be undertaken for all people on admission to residential care facilities.
- Mobility – frail elderly people may be house or bed-bound and unable to travel to a dental surgery for care. This requires domiciliary care. Here, the dentist travels to the patient, as opposed to the more usual patient coming to see the dentist.
- Mobile dental equipment – improved equipment, including high-torque handpieces, makes bedside care more feasible.
- Difficulty tolerating treatment.
- Lack of mental capacity and the need to adhere to legal requirements to ensure consent is valid and treatment is in the patient's best interest when they lack understanding of their own care needs.
- Co-morbidity:
  - dental problems may have an impact on general health
  - general health, and the medications used to treat problems, may have an impact on oral health.
- Many care homes have arrangements with local general dental practitioners to provide care for their residents, but frequently, these are on an independent/private basis rather than via the National Health Service. Some community dental services have established managed clinical networks to administer domiciliary care.

- Social enterprise companies are a possible means of addressing the provision of dental care to care homes.

Homeless people

The homeless are those who lack permanent accommodation. Homeless people may be living in temporary accommodation, bed-and-breakfast establishments or hostels, 'sofa-surfing', staying with friends or sleeping rough. In late 2022, there were 72,550 households assessed as homeless or threatened with homelessness. A census in autumn 2022 estimated that in England, just over 3000 people were sleeping rough each night. Access to healthcare is a significant issue for people who are homeless. Surveys show that access to dental care comes high on the list of health needs of people living on the streets.

Issues include:
- Levels of decay and tooth loss are higher than in the general population
- Older homeless people are frequently edentulous and do not have dentures
- Homeless people lack social and supportive contacts
- Mental health issues compound other problems
- Addiction to alcohol and drugs is common, leading to further dental health problems.

Gypsies and Travellers

Gypsies and Travellers are a specific cultural group who are vulnerable and frequently experience difficulty in accessing dental care. Data on their oral health needs are limited to non-existent. This group is frequently invisible to Commissioners, not only in relation to oral health but health in general.

Issues include:
- They frequently live in overcrowded and less than satisfactory accommodation
- Levels of disease are higher, and life expectancy is lower than in the general population
- Cultural beliefs affect their trust in health professionals
- They face racism and prejudice
- Their access to healthcare is problematic
- Their levels of general literacy and health literacy are low.

Substance misusers

The following issues have impacts on oral health and dental care for people who are addicted to drugs and alcohol:
- They experience high levels of dental caries, which is untreated
- Their chaotic lifestyle prevents routine dental attendance, and they may fail to keep appointments
- Patients are likely to present in acute dental pain
- Patients may have significant health problems, such as blood-borne virus infection or mental health issues
- Addicts may demand opiate-based analgesics, e.g. codeine
- Methadone, used in heroin-replacement therapy programmes, is cariogenic due to its high sugar content – the sugar-free variety should be encouraged.

Other groups

Two specific groups who have special arrangements for the provision of dental care are prisoners and the armed forces. Issues related to these groups are shown in Boxes 36.2 and 36.3.

37 Screening and diagnostic tests

Figure 37.1 The parameters that can be calculated to determine the value of a screening or diagnostic test

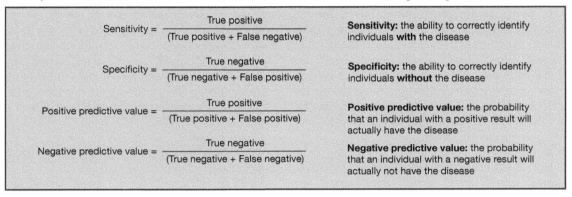

$$\text{Sensitivity} = \frac{\text{True positive}}{(\text{True positive} + \text{False negative})}$$

Sensitivity: the ability to correctly identify individuals **with** the disease

$$\text{Specificity} = \frac{\text{True negative}}{(\text{True negative} + \text{False positive})}$$

Specificity: the ability to correctly identify individuals **without** the disease

$$\text{Positive predictive value} = \frac{\text{True positive}}{(\text{True positive} + \text{False positive})}$$

Positive predictive value: the probability that an individual with a positive result will actually have the disease

$$\text{Negative predictive value} = \frac{\text{True negative}}{(\text{True negative} + \text{False negative})}$$

Negative predictive value: the probability that an individual with a negative result will actually not have the disease

Figure 37.2 Diagrammatic representation of a receiver operating diagnostic (ROC) curve

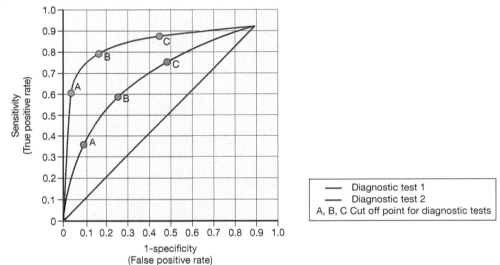

Sensitivity (True positive rate) vs 1-specificity (False positive rate)

— Diagnostic test 1
— Diagnostic test 2
A, B, C Cut off point for diagnostic tests

Table 37.1 Criteria for the establishment of a screening programme

Criteria	Considerations
Is the disease an important health issue?	The prevalence and impact of the disease require consideration.
Is the screening test acceptable to patients?	If the screening test is overly burdensome or in some way is not acceptable to the majority of the population to be screened, uptake will be low, and the programme will be ineffective.
Is there a recognisable latent or early symptomatic stage?	There is little point in screening for a disease that will, at an early stage, become evident and lead the patient to seek care due to signs and symptoms.
Are facilities for diagnosis and treatment available?	A positive screen will require the resources to undertake a definitive diagnostic test and to treat patients confirmed as having the disease.
Has the opportunity cost been considered?	Spending money and resources on a screening programme means that these resources are not available to use for an alternative intervention.
Is there an agreed policy on who to treat as patients?	This means is it clear when an individual has the disease and when not – is a definitive diagnosis possible?
Does treatment confer benefit?	This raises the question of whether there is any material advantage to the patient in identifying their disease earlier than would otherwise be the case. If knowing the patient has the disease early results in a better health outcome, then clearly screening is advantageous. However, if there is no difference in treatment outcome as a result of early diagnosis, then a screening programme may add unnecessarily to costs and result in patients having longer knowledge of the disease with no material benefit and the possible worry of knowing they have the disease and being labelled as a patient.

Source: *Wilson and Junger (1968). Reproduced with permission from the World Health Organization.*

Dental Public Health at a Glance, Second Edition. Ivor G. Chestnutt.
© 2024 John Wiley & Sons Ltd. Published 2024 by John Wiley & Sons Ltd.

Screening

Screening in the context of public health programmes is usually designed to enable early diagnosis of a disease or condition.

Screening implies the systematic application of a test or procedure to a population perceived to be at risk of the disease of interest.

Examples of screening programmes in the United Kingdom are the range of tests applied to all newborn babies to detect metabolic disorders and programmes to detect breast and cervical cancer in women and bowel cancer in both men and women. There are no formal national screening programmes for oral disease.

Screening versus diagnosis

It is very important to understand the difference between screening and diagnosis. Screening aims to identify those who are likely to have the disease in question. A positive screening test does not always imply that the individual has the disease. Furthermore, more definitive or invasive tests are often required to confirm a diagnosis. So, in the case of screening for bowel cancer, a positive occult blood sample in a stool sample requires further investigation to determine whether cancer is present.

Criteria for the establishment of a screening programme

There are a number of criteria that need to be satisfied before a screening programme is implemented (Table 37.1).

Oral cancer

Recommendations on the implementation of a screening programme for a given disease are made by the United Kingdom National Screening Committee. When oral cancer was last reviewed, the Committee concluded that systematic population screening was not justified. Instead, the current practice is for dental professionals to undertake opportunistic screening.

Dental caries

For most of the twentieth century, the Community Dental Service (and its predecessor, the School Dental Service) undertook 'school dental screening', and there was a statutory obligation to do so. While this process was called screening, it was, in fact, a diagnosis. The objective of the exercise was to identify children who had untreated dental decay and who were not under the care of a dentist and to inform parents of their child's oral status. In the latter part of the twentieth century, the effectiveness of mass screening of school children for dental decay was questioned. The main issue was, once the need was identified, ensuring that parents subsequently took their children to the dentist. The role of the Community Dental Service changed from routine care of children to focussing on looking after those with special needs. This has led to traditional school screening being abandoned in most areas.

The value of a screening or diagnostic test

The application of a diagnostic or screening test can have four possible outcomes, as shown in Table 37.2. The usefulness of a screening or diagnostic test is dependent on the proportion of individuals who have the disease and are correctly identified as having the disease in question (sensitivity) and the proportion of individuals who do not have the disease and are correctly identified as not having the disease (specificity); see Figure 37.1. Clearly, it is desirable to have both of these proportions as high as possible. They are influenced by the cut-off point for the screening or diagnostic test in question. Increasing the cut-off point to increase the sensitivity of test results in a decrease in its specificity. So, setting up the test to increase the proportion of people who are correctly tested as positive means that there is a trade-off in the number of individuals correctly identified as not having the disease.

Receiver operating characteristic (ROC) curves

The usefulness of a screening or diagnostic test can be demonstrated visually by plotting a receiver operating characteristic (ROC) curve, as shown in Figure 37.2.

Examples of the use of ROC curves in dentistry include the evaluation of tests determining caries risk in children; histological validation of cone-beam computed tomography versus laser fluorescence and conventional diagnostic methods for occlusal caries detection; and validating screening methods for periodontitis using salivary haemoglobin level and self-report questionnaires in disabled people.

The sensitivity (true positive rate) is plotted against 1-sensitivity (the false positive rate) for different cut-off points used to define positive and negative in the test (e.g. points A, B and C in Figure 37.2). A diagonal line is drawn at 45° through the origin. The area under the curve to this line relates to the performance of the test. So, the further the curve approaches the top left of the graph, the better the test. In Figure 37.2, Test 1 (red line) has greater utility (i.e. is better at correctly identifying positives and negatives) than Test 2 (blue line).

Table 37.2 The possible outcomes from the application of a screening or diagnostic test

Test result	Disease status	
	Has the disease	Does not have the disease
Positive	True positive	False positive
Negative	False negative	True negative

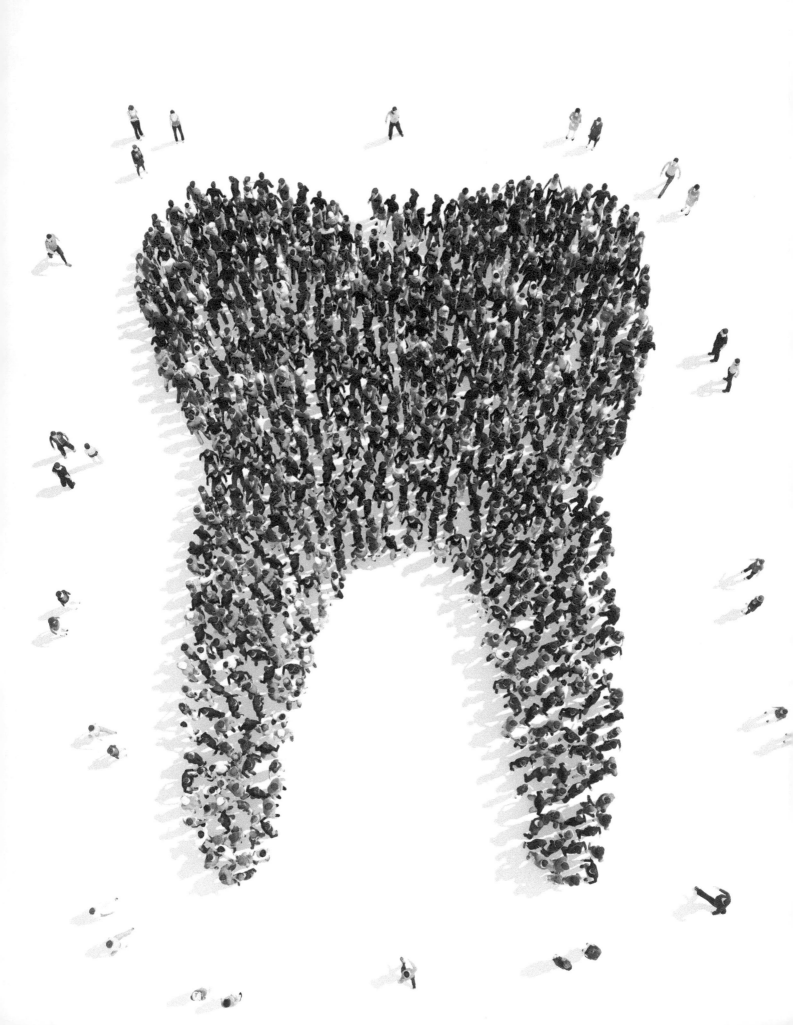

Providing dental services

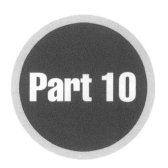

Part 10

Chapters

38 Health economics

Table 38.1 Approaches to health economic analysis

When to use	Dental example	Notes
Cost-minimisation analysis		
Cost-minimisation analysis is used when the health outcomes of two or more interventions are the same or similar in all important aspects – and have been shown to be so in a clinical trial.	This type of analysis would be suitable to evaluate the use of two mouthwashes that resulted in the same level of dental plaque reduction and had similar side-effect profiles. It could be used in comparing a branded product with a generic version of the same product. The least costly option would be that of choice.	This a simple technique, but it requires the data to confirm that the clinical and side-effect outcomes are the same.
Cost–utility analysis		
Cost–utility analysis compares different interventions with varying health outcomes. The common 'currency' of a utility measure, most commonly a QUALY, is used to compare outcomes.	This type of analysis would be suitable to evaluate different approaches to the treatment of head and neck cancer.	It is necessary to define and measure the health states of interest. The utility can be considered either from the perspective of individual patients or society. Techniques for eliciting utility values include: • Standard gamble • Time trade-off • Visual analogue or rating scale.
Cost-effectiveness analysis		
Cost-effectiveness analysis is used when the health benefits of interventions are measured in natural units, reflecting a dominant common therapeutic goal for different therapies.	This type of analysis could be used to compare the relative merits of fissure sealants and fluoride varnish in preventing new caries lesions on the occlusal surfaces of teeth. Here, the unit of analysis is the number of carious surfaces avoided.	Results would be presented in the form of how much it costs to prevent an additional tooth surface from becoming carious (incremental cost). The different interventions are compared by determining the cost-effectiveness ratio. This is calculated by dividing the cost of the intervention by the health effect outcome. This is the most common type of health economic analysis reported in the literature.
Cost–benefit analysis		
Cost–benefit analysis is used when both costs and benefits are measured in monetary units. The financial value of the costs is compared with the financial benefits of the interventions.	Cost–benefit analysis has been used to determine the economic impact of water fluoridation.	The intervention is deemed favourable when the financial value of the benefits is in excess of the financial value of the costs. This approach does not take into account quality-of-life measurements and thus is unable to account for different patient groups with different outcome measures. This approach informs value for money and can guide priority setting.

Table 38.2 Types of economic analysis and subject investigated in a review of 33 economic evaluations on oral health preventive programmes

Type of economic analysis	No of studies	Topic investigated	No of studies
Cost-effectiveness analysis (CEA)	24	Sealants and varnishes	13
Cost utility analysis (CUA)	4	Water fluoridation	3
Cost benefit analysis	1	Other caries preventive programmes	5
Combination of CEA and CUA	4	Periodontal disease prevention	2
		Oral cancer screening	4
		Other topics inc. the management of third molars	6

Source: *Data from Mariño et al. (2020). Quality appraisal of economic evaluations done on oral health preventive programs-A systematic review Journal of Public Health Dentistry. https://doi.org/10.1111/jphd.12368.*

Health economics

Health economics deals with a scarcity of resources and the clinical effectiveness and cost-effectiveness of healthcare provision. Health economic analysis informs how maximum value can be achieved from available resources.

Maximising outcomes from scarce resources

The resources available to provide healthcare, whether viewed from the perspective of an individual, a health insurance company or a government, are finite. The potential needs for and potential to benefit from healthcare are infinite. In the United Kingdom, the population is increasing in number and ageing. Medical and dental technology is ever-expanding in both scope and complexity. Society and those who make decisions on its behalf, therefore, face the difficult decision of how the defined resources available are best used to achieve the optimum outcome.

Typical decisions facing politicians, health policymakers and clinicians are as follows. If a new drug for treating cancer costs £40,000 per patient cared for, is that a better use of the money than providing joint replacements costing £10,000 each for four patients? In coming to a decision on this matter, it is necessary not only to consider the number of patients treated, but the clinical outcome and the quality of life resulting for the patients concerned. If the cancer drug extends the patient's life by 6 months, but the joint replacement relieves pain, increases mobility and lasts for 10 years, which is the better use of the £40,000?

These are the types of questions that health economics helps answer because resources are always scarce. This means that both the clinical effectiveness and cost-effectiveness of interventions have to be considered when planning and commissioning resources. The following concepts are important in health economics.

Clinical effectiveness

As is evident from the name, clinical effectiveness relates to the clinical/health outcome of an intervention. It is about what works and is central to the concept of evidence-based practice (Chapter 18).

Cost-effectiveness

Cost-effectiveness implies either a desire to achieve a predetermined objective at least cost or a desire to maximise the benefit to the population of patients served from a limited amount of resources.

Efficiency

Efficiency evaluates how well resources are used to achieve a desired outcome.

Utility measures

Utility is defined as the level of satisfaction that consumers derive from having their desires met. In the context of health economics, it relates to preferences for different health states. Utility measures have two dimensions – a quantitative dimension, which measures enhanced survival (years added to life), and a qualitative dimension, which accounts for the quality of life (QoL, life added to years). Quality of life is assessed using components such as the ability to perform the functions of daily living, presence of pain and mental disturbance.

Quality-adjusted life years (QALYs)

The years added to life by a health intervention and the quality of life during those years are combined to produce quality-adjusted life years (QALYs). This reflects the number of years lived in a given health state. QALYs are presented as a value between 0 and 1, where 0 = death and 1 = one year of life in perfect health. A score less than 0 would indicate a health state worse than death. The advantage of this approach is that it allows health interventions with different clinical outcomes to be compared, as in the example of the new cancer drug and the provision of joint replacements given earlier.

The costs of different health interventions can be expressed as the cost per QALY gained. For publicly funded health interventions, the National Institute for Health and Care Excellence (NICE) currently values one QALY at between £20,000 and £30,000.

QALYs and oral health

The application of analysis using QALYs to oral health interventions is problematic, as dental procedures generally are not directly life-lengthening. The concept of quality-adjusted tooth years (QATYs), where a missing tooth would score 0 and a sound functioning tooth would score 1, has been proposed, but has not been used to any great degree.

Types of health economic evaluation

There are four common types of economic evaluation:
- Cost-minimization analysis
- Cost–utility analysis
- Cost-effectiveness analysis
- Cost–benefit analysis

These are described in Table 38.1. The frequency with which these analyses are described in the economic analysis of caries-prevention programmes is shown in Table 38.2.

Capital and recurrent costs

In health service planning, costs are described as capital and recurrent. Capital costs are one-off costs that are not directly linked to output. Typical examples are equipment, for instance, a dental chair, an autoclave, or a new surgery. Recurrent costs, as the name suggests, represent expenditure that is repeated and ongoing, such as staff salaries, materials, costs of using equipment such as electricity and annual service charges.

In any healthcare system, staff costs (salaries) are usually the largest item of expenditure.

Opportunity costs

Because resources are finite, there is an opportunity cost to all decisions in healthcare. This means that if we decide to undertake activity x, then we are required to forego activity y. For example, if a dental practice owner decides to spend one hour each month holding a staff meeting, that time cannot be used to see and treat patients. The opportunity cost of the meeting is reduced patient throughput. However, in the interests of an efficiently run and safe practice, it is likely that the benefit of the staff meeting will outweigh not treating patients during that one-hour session and the reduction in income that results.

39 How the National Health Service is organised

Figure 39.1 The structure of the NHS in England. Source: *Reproduced from House of Commons Library, 2023 / National Health Service / Public Domain CC BY 3.0.*

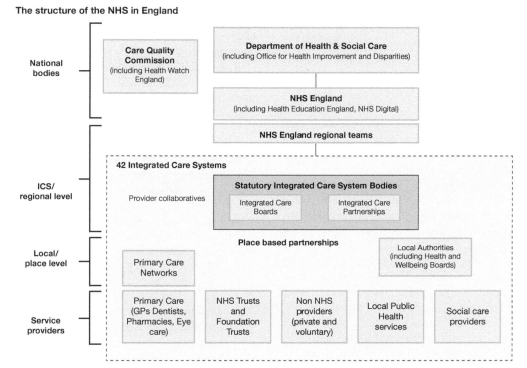

Figure 39.2 Integrated Care Systems (ICSs): key planning and partnership bodies from July 2022. Source: *The King's Fund with permission.*

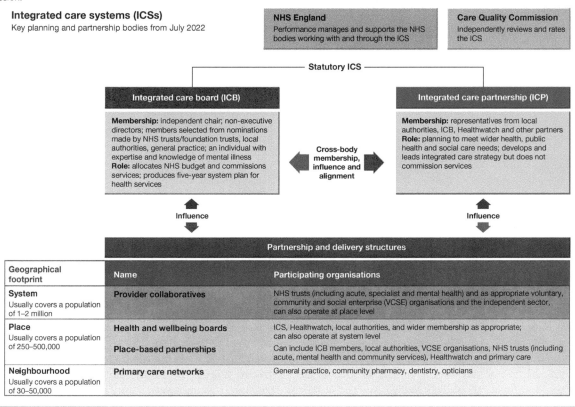

Dental Public Health at a Glance, Second Edition. Ivor G. Chestnutt.
© 2024 John Wiley & Sons Ltd. Published 2024 by John Wiley & Sons Ltd.

Health services across the United Kingdom

In 1999, following public referenda, governments were established in Scotland and Wales in addition to the existing administration in Northern Ireland. This process was known as devolution. Whilst some aspects of national life, such as defence services, remained under the control of the central United Kingdom Government in London, others including responsibility for the provision of health services, were transferred to the parliaments in Edinburgh, Cardiff and Belfast.

Since 1999, how health services are commissioned and delivered has diverged markedly in the constituent countries of the UK. These differences also apply to how public health is organised and how dental care is commissioned.

The NHS in England

Political direction

Overall health policy is directed by the government of the day via the Department of Health and Social Care (DHSC).

NHS England

NHS England, an arm's length body of the DHSC, is responsible for the commissioning of health services and allocating the budget from the government to different parts of the NHS (Figure 39.1).

Integrated Care Systems

The Health and Social Care Act 2022 made extensive changes to the structure of the NHS in England. The Act established 42 Integrated Care Systems (ICSs) across England. These took on statutory responsibility for most local NHS services on 1 July 2022. ICSs are also responsible for improving the health of the local population, and for integrating health and social care services.

Within ICSs, a range of local arrangements exist to plan and deliver joined-up services. These include 'place-based partnerships' and primary care networks, which are groups of GP practices. These partnerships and networks also involve community, mental health, social care and hospital services working together (Figure 39.2).

In carrying out their responsibilities, NHS England and integrated care boards are subject to statutory duties, including:
- promoting the NHS Constitution
- securing continuous improvements in the quality of services commissioned
- reducing inequalities
- enabling choice and promoting patient involvement
- securing integration
- promoting innovation and research.

Care Quality Commission

The Care Quality Commission (CQC) is responsible for the registration, inspection and monitoring of health and adult social care services, including both NHS and independent providers. This includes dental providers (Chapter 50).

National Institute for Health and Care Excellence

The National Institute for Health and Care Excellence (NICE) is an independent body that provides evidence-based guidance on health services, social care and public health (Chapter 18).

Public health services

The Health and Social Care Act 2012 transferred responsibility for a range of public health services from the NHS to local authorities, and a Director of Public Health is responsible for leading public health responsibilities within a local authority. This change reflects the fact that the determinants of health are much wider than simply those that are the responsibility of health services (e.g. environment, housing, leisure facilities, education) (Chapter 2).

Some aspects of public health services, such as the national immunisation and national screening programmes, are provided directly by NHS England.

United Kingdom Health Security Agency (UKHSA)

This agency replaced Public Health England. It has a UK-wide role in protecting against infectious diseases and external health threats.

Issues facing the National Health Service across the United Kingdom

The NHS celebrated its 75th Anniversary in 2023. However, the service is facing a number of issues that put pressure on how it operates to deliver effective and efficient services. These include:
- An ageing population
- A growing population
- Advances in the technical complexity and cost of treatments and drugs
- Workforce issues relating to training, recruitment and retention of suitably trained staff
- The impact of Brexit and the UK's exit from the European Union
- The disruption caused by the COVID-19 pandemic when the service had to deal with many seriously ill patients, the impact of the pandemic on staff, the suspension of routine care during the pandemic and the backlog of patients awaiting routine care that has resulted and the service has struggled to manage
- Lack of capacity in social care services, which results in difficulty discharging from hospital patients who are 'medically fit for discharge' but who require social care, which isn't available
- Finance – austerity measures, inefficiencies in the service, rising inflation after a decade of low inflation, and staff pay issues are all impacting on how the NHS operates across the UK
- Constant changes in how the service is structured as dictated when governments change and even whilst the same party remains in power
- Political views on how much service should be contracted out to the private sector.

How dental care is organised in the United Kingdom

Table 40.1 Definitions and examples of primary, secondary and tertiary care

Primary care – services that patients can access directly, e.g. General Dental Service, Community Dental Service, General Medical Service, opticians, pharmacists.
Secondary care – services that patients can access only on referral by a primary care practitioner, e.g. most hospital services, specialist NHS dental services.
Tertiary care – specialist services to which referrals are made by secondary care services, e.g. cleft lip and palate services.

Table 40.2 The number of registrants on the General Dental Council Specialist Lists in the United Kingdom, December 2022

Specialty	Number of practitioners on the list
Dental and Maxillofacial Radiology	31
Dental Public Health	88
Endodontics	321
Oral and Maxillofacial Pathology	35
Oral Medicine	66
Oral Microbiology	6
Oral Surgery	749
Orthodontics	1395
Paediatric Dentistry	251
Periodontics	395
Prosthodontics	453
Restorative Dentistry	300
Special Care Dentistry	277
Total	**4367**

Source: *General Dental Council, Registration Statistical Report (2022).*

Healthcare is defined as being primary, secondary or tertiary (Table 40.1).

Primary dental care

General Dental Service (GDS)

The majority of dental care (85%) is provided in primary care by general dental practitioners (GDPs). GDPs are independent practitioners who contract with the National Health Service (NHS) to provide an agreed volume of dental care. In England, practitioners contract with NHS England. In Wales, Scotland, and Northern Ireland, dentists contract with local Health Boards. Traditionally,

GDS was provided by one or two dentists working from dental practices in the high street, often in buildings originally built for a purpose other than the provision of dental care. Increasingly, GDS services are provided from multi-surgery, purpose-built premises and the contract may be held by a corporate body (company). In these circumstances, the dentist, dental hygienist or dental therapist is often employed on a salaried basis.

Community/Salaried/Public Dental Services (CDS)

These services provide dental care for people whose social, medical and dental needs mean they cannot be efficiently and effectively managed in the General Dental Service. Dental staff working in the CDS are salaried employees of the NHS. The CDS evolved from the School Dental Service in the mid-1970s. The degree to which it continues to act as a safety net service for high-need children in areas of social and economic deprivation varies across the United Kingdom. The CDS nowadays looks after elderly and housebound people and those with severe physical disabilities or mental illnesses.

In addition to the provision of care to high-need groups, the CDS provides staff who undertake local and national epidemiological studies of oral health. It is also responsible for delivering oral health promotion and education programmes and is intimately involved in national oral health improvement programmes such as Childsmile and Designed to Smile.

In Scotland, the CDS is known as the Public Dental Service, while in England, the term Salaried Dental Service is used.

Personal Dental Service (PDS)

This form of dental service allows for variation in the standard GDS and CDS commissioning arrangements and is used to procure specific types of service, such as domiciliary care or sedation services.

Secondary dental care

Hospital Dental Services (HDS)

Hospital dental services provide specialist dental care, either from general hospitals or from one of the dedicated dental hospitals. The most commonly provided services are oral and maxillofacial surgery and orthodontics. In dental hospitals, the full range of dental specialist services is provided, including restorative dentistry, oral radiology and oral microbiology. Dental hospitals, in conjunction with a local university also have responsibility for training the next generation of dental professionals.

Specialist dental care

It is possible for patients to access specialist dental care directly, usually outside the NHS, on a private patient basis. Dentists who have undertaken additional specialist training and are registered on Specialist Lists held by the General Dental Council (GDC) may describe themselves as specialists and offer services directly to the public. Such practitioners often also take referrals from colleagues in the GDS and provide treatments that are either too complex, for example, oral surgery, or prohibitively expensive to provide under the GDS, for instance, advanced endodontics or dental implants. Dental practitioners must not mislead patients into thinking that they possess additional specialist skills unless they are registered as a specialist with the GDC.

Specialist lists

Specialist lists, held by the General Dental Council are made up of registered dentists who meet certain conditions and so are entitled to use a specialist title. Dentists do not have to join a specialist list to practise any particular specialty but they can only use the title 'specialist' if they are on that list.

Specialist lists are designed to:
• protect the public against unwarranted claims of specialist skills and experience
• help the public, employers and others identify dentists with recognised specialist skills and experience in a distinct branch of dentistry and to support appropriate patient referral
• support the development of scientific knowledge and education.

The specialties recognised by the General Dental Council are shown in Table 40.2.

NHS and independent (private) dental care

The GDS, CDS and HDS provide care under the NHS. In addition, a substantial proportion of dental care is provided independently of the NHS. This enables patients to access routine care and care that is not provided under the NHS, such as cosmetic treatments or advanced restorative procedures. As independent contractors, GDPs may opt to provide all of their care independently, or to undertake mixed practice whereby they devote some of their time to providing care under an NHS contract and some outside the NHS. Care must be taken to ensure that patients are fully aware from the outset of the arrangements under which their care is being provided.

Patient involvement in dental care

In the past, healthcare professionals were seen as the possessors of wisdom and knowledge and largely instructed patients as to what they saw as being in the patient's best interests. Thankfully, this attitude has changed, and patients can now expect to be fully informed and involved in decisions about the options for their care. Dental professionals have a responsibility to ensure that their patients are fully appraised of all treatment options, the benefits, risks, consequences and costs of these options, before embarking on a course of treatment.

Commissioning NHS Dental Services

In England, the responsibility for commissioning (contracting for) dental services lies with NHS England via their Integrated Care Boards (from September 2023) via local area teams. In Scotland and Wales, the commissioning of NHS dental care lies with Health Boards. In Northern Ireland, the Strategic Planning and Performance Group of the Department of Health and Social Care oversees contracts with dental practitioners.

In September 2003, the priorities of NHS Dental Commissioners in England were:
• To reduce oral health inequalities and improve oral health in children under the age of five
• Flexible commissioning
• To oversee national dental access and address areas of weakest dental provision
• To ensure a consistent and fair approach to contract performance management is applied nationally to dental contracts
• Dental contract reform.

41 Paying for dental care

Table 41.1 Advantages and disadvantages of different systems of paying for dental services

Payment system	Fee per item	Capitation	Salary
Advantages	Provider paid for each item of treatment provided Provider incentivised to treat all existing disease	Commissioner can control costs more easily Allows both provider and commissioner to plan and budget more easily Advantageous to providers in low dental need patients	Beneficial when treating patients who require specialist care/whose treatment needs are more time-consuming Allows the commissioner to plan and budget more easily
Disadvantages	Risks overtreatment More difficult for commissioners to control costs	Risks of undertreatment (supervised neglect) Potentially disadvantageous to providers in areas of high dental need	Without effective management, risks being inefficient

Table 41.2 Courses of treatment in the England and Wales NHS dental service (bands), their respective values (units of dental activity) and patient co-payments

Course of treatment	Treatment included	Units of dental activity[a]	Charge to non-exempt patients, NHS England (2023 prices)[b]
Band 1	Examination, scale and polish, radiographs and preventive treatments	1	£25.80
Band 2	Treatments in Band 1 plus restorations, root fillings and extractions	3	£70.70
Modifications to Band 2 treatments in England from Nov 2022			
Band 2a	Covers all Band 2 treatments other than Band 2b and Band 2c.	3	
Band 2b	Covers a course of treatment involving either non-molar endodontics to permanent teeth or a combined total of three or more teeth requiring permanent fillings or extractions.	5	
Band 2c	Covers a course of treatment involving molar endodontics on permanent teeth.	7	
Band 3	Treatments in Bands 1 and 2 plus crowns, bridges and dentures	12	£306.80
Urgent	Relief of pain/arrest of haemorrhage	1.2	As Band 1

[a] The average price paid per UDA to dentists by the NHS is £25 (2022).
[b] Patient charges in Wales are less than those levied in England.

Table 41.3 Public dental service entitlement and arrangements for patient co-payments in selected countries

Country	Population covered	Patient co-payment
Australia	Targeted groups only: adults on low incomes, those with chronic conditions or complex care needs, children and adolescents	Some dental services provided to eligible groups attract user charges, including school dental services; user charges vary regionally/locally
Canada	Targeted groups only: indigenous people, armed forces, refugees, local and provincial programmes (e.g. for individuals on low incomes)	Dental services provided to eligible user groups may attract user charges; these vary regionally/locally
England	Universal entitlement	Patients who are not exempt on the grounds of being <18 years old, pregnant or nursing mother, receiving income-related benefit, pay one of three charges dependent on the complexity of the course of treatment
Finland	Universal entitlement	User charges are determined locally within limits set by the government; patients contribute 20% of costs on average
France	Universal entitlement under social health insurance	Social health insurance covers 70% of the costs of healthcare, including dental services; the remaining 30% is paid by the patient
Germany	Entitlement under social health insurance (covering about 88% of the population)	Some patient co-payments are required – up to 50% in the case of crowns. bridges and dentures
Netherlands	Universal entitlement to a basic package of health services	Patients pay 25% of the cost of prostheses
New Zealand	Targeted groups only: individuals on low incomes or with complex care needs	Patients make a contribution to emergency dental care
Spain	Universal entitlement to acute dental care – more comprehensive treatment for children, pregnant women, disabled people and pensioners	Public dental services do not involve user charges
Sweden	Universal entitlement	Patients contribute to the cost of treatment on a sliding scale

Dental Public Health at a Glance, Second Edition. Ivor G. Chestnutt.
© 2024 John Wiley & Sons Ltd. Published 2024 by John Wiley & Sons Ltd.

Mechanisms of paying for dental care

There are three principal mechanisms of paying for dental care:

- **Fee per item:** Where a charge is made for each item of treatment provided.
- **Capitation:** Where the providing dentist receives a lump sum to provide care for a set number of patients.
- **Salary:** Where the providing dentist is paid a salary to provide care.

There are advantages and disadvantages to each of these payment systems (Table 41.1). They can be viewed from the perspective of both the provider of care (dental professional) and the commissioner of care (the NHS, insurance company or patient).

Current mechanisms of paying for dental care

National Health Service

The payment mechanism used varies across the United Kingdom. Over the last three decades, several different payment systems have been employed in an attempt to ensure the effective and efficient provision of NHS dental care. Traditionally, NHS dentistry was based on a fee-per-item system of payment, and this is still the main basis of payments to NHS GDS dentists in Scotland and Northern Ireland. In England and Wales, arrangements are based on a system where dentists' output is measured in units of dental activity (UDA), and care is divided into three bands. This system, which was introduced in 2006, is widely recognised as flawed. The main drawback is the insensitivity to gradations of patient needs. Under the UDA system, until recently, a dentist was paid the same fee for a patient who requires four restorations as for a patient who requires only one restoration (both qualified as Band 2 treatments). In recognition of this major limitation, Band 2 treatments in England were expanded, as shown in Table 41.2. Dentists contract with NHS England or with the local Health Board in Wales (Chapter 40) to provide a specified number of UDAs on an annual basis. The clinical activity that falls within each of the three treatment bands, the UDAs that can be claimed and the patient co-payment are shown in Table 41.2. Currently, contract reform is underway in England and Wales in an attempt to devise a more equitable way of contracting for state funded primary dental care services.

Patient co-payments

To offset the costs of NHS dental care, patients are required to make a co-payment. In England and Wales, this is one of three fees that relate to the treatment band provided in any course of treatment (Table 41.2). In Scotland, patients pay 80% of the cost of their treatment up to a maximum of £384 per course of treatment (2022/2023 cost).

Those aged under 18 years, under 19 years and in full-time education, women who are pregnant or have had a baby in the past 12 months and those in receipt of Income Support or income-related benefits are exempt from NHS patient charges.

At the time of writing, alternative ways of providing and paying for NHS dental care in England and Wales are being piloted.

Dental professionals working in Hospital and Community Dental Services are paid a salary. Normally, there is no patient co-charge for care provided in these settings, although, in some circumstances, charges are levied for prostheses.

Independent (private) dental care

Patients can either pay their dental provider directly on a fee-per-item basis or join a dental insurance scheme, such as Denplan or BUPA. Typically, for the latter the patient will pay a set monthly fee (which will vary according to their risk of future dental problems judged by their past treatment). This fee covers routine check-up examinations and basic care. Additional payments may be required if patients subsequently need more advanced restorative procedures such as crowns, bridges or implants.

Payment for dental services – International perspective

In the United Kingdom, very few individuals will have dental insurance provided by their employer. However, in the United States, employer-provided dental insurance is how most patients pay for their dental care. This means that those who are not employed or employed in a low-grade job will not have dental insurance. American children who are enroled in the Medicaid programme are technically entitled to dental care – although the availability of willing dental care providers is a problem. While individual states are mandated to provide dental care for children, the provision of dental care for adults under the Medicaid programme is left to the state's discretion. Although most provide access to emergency dental care, less than half currently provide comprehensive dental coverage for poor and disadvantaged citizens.

In other countries, the provision of Public Dental Services varies in relation to the proportion of the population covered and the degree to which patients must contribute towards the cost of their care. The position in some selected countries is illustrated in Table 41.3.

A blended dental contract

Given the pros and cons of different mechanisms of paying for public dental services, it is likely that an optimal system would involve a 'blended contract' whereby dentists receive a proportion of their income from capitation, allowances and a fee per item. This should be modelled to take into account the varying needs of the population served and the level of care that the commissioning body (that is, the government in the case of publicly funded services) wishes to provide. However, such a model is complex to devise and administer.

Barriers to accessing dental care

Figure 42.1 Self-reported frequency of attendance for 'routine dental check-up' by adults in Wales, 2019. Source: *Public Health Wales.*

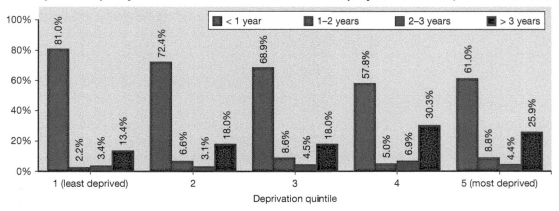

Figure 42.2 Potential barriers to accessing dental care

Patient related factors
- Perceived need
- Fatalistic attitude
- Lack of awareness
- Anxiety/fear
- Past dental experiences
- Disability – mental and/or physical
- Time availability – getting time off work
- Ethnic and cultural beliefs and practices

Dentist related factors
- Professional attitude
- Perceived competence of dentist by patients
- Availability of dentists with specialist skills

System related factors
- Cost
- Availability of NHS services
- Physical barriers – e.g. surgery accessible only via steps/stairs
- Rural and remote area issues
- Availability of transport

Table 42.1 Different types of need using dental attendance as an example

Need	Definition
Normative needs	Defined by experts, e.g. the frequency with which dental professionals recommend visiting a dentist
Felt needs	Those needs people say they have, e.g. a patient's description of how often they wish to visit a dentist
Expressed needs	Needs expressed by action, e.g. visiting a dentist
Comparative needs	Comparing one group of people with another, e.g. comparing dental attendance of different groups in relation to social and economic deprivation

Source: *Adapted from Bradshaw (1972).*

Dental Public Health at a Glance, Second Edition. Ivor G. Chestnutt.
© 2024 John Wiley & Sons Ltd. Published 2024 by John Wiley & Sons Ltd.

There are a number of barriers that may prevent a patient from accessing dental care either at all or as often as they need to or wish to.

Frequency of dental attendance

Guidance from the National Institute for Health and Care Excellence (NICE) recommends that recall intervals be based on disease risk and vary between 3 and 24 months in adults. A survey of adults in Wales in 2019 prior to the COVID-19 pandemic demonstrated that over two-thirds of the survey participants (67.3%) reported that they had visited a dentist for a dental 'check-up' (NHS, private or mixed) within the previous 12 months. However, 21.8% had not had a dental 'check-up' for more than three years. As deprivation increased, the proportion of survey participants who had been to a dentist for a routine dental 'check-up' within the previous 12 months decreased (most deprived = 61.0%; least deprived = 81.0%). In contrast, 25.9% and 30.3% of people living in the most deprived and next deprived quintile areas, respectively, reported that they had not had a dental 'check-up' for more than three years (Figure 42.1).

Successive epidemiological surveys show that women attend the dentist more regularly than men. Just 2% of adults claimed never to have attended a dentist.

Barriers to dental care

Perceptions of need

In order for patients to attend for care, they must feel or perceive the need to attend. Need can be viewed from different perspectives. It should be recognised that the perceptions of dental professionals and patients may differ when discussing the need for dental attendance. Definitions of need are shown in Table 42.1.

Patient attitudes as a barrier to care

Around a quarter of the population attends the dentist sporadically or only when provoked by a problem. This may reflect a lack of awareness of need, a fatalistic attitude or anxiety and fears about dental attendance.

Anxiety about dental attendance can be measured using the Modified Dental Anxiety Scale. This simple questionnaire asks potential patients to rate how worried they would be about attending the dentist and the types of procedures they might undergo during a dental appointment. In the 2009 Adult Dental Health Survey, 30% of adults said that having a tooth drilled would make them very or extremely anxious, and 28% reported similar levels of anxiety about having a local anaesthetic.

Costs as a barrier to care

The cost of dental care can be a barrier. This has been shown to prevent patients from attending the dentist, to prevent patients from having the treatment they would like and to cause patients to delay or put off having treatment.

While the NHS dental system in the United Kingdom exempts patients who are receiving Income Support from co-payments (Chapter 41), in any means-tested system, there are always those who just fail to qualify for welfare payments but for whom the cost of dental care may be a burden. The 'cost-of-living crisis' experienced in 2022/2023 in the aftermath of the COVID-19 pandemic and the geopolitical uncertainties arising from Russian's illegal invasion of Ukraine has impacted what people can and cannot afford. This may well affect people's decisions on dental attendance or the affordability of care they might need/desire.

Dental professionals should make clear the costs of dental care at the commencement of treatment, and the General Dental Council requires that patients be given a written treatment plan with details of costs before treatment is carried out. The onus to be clear about costs lies with the dental team. Patients have reported that it may not be the actual cost that is the issue, but concerns over not knowing the cost and embarrassment about raising this issue when vulnerable in the dental chair that forms the real barrier. Dentistry is one of the few areas of healthcare in the United Kingdom where patients have to pay at the point of delivery, and so patients may lack the confidence and skills to enquire about and negotiate costs, especially if paying directly out of their own pocket rather than via a dental insurance scheme.

Increasingly patients desire treatments that are primarily for cosmetic purposes, such as tooth whitening or adult orthodontics, which may not be available via state-funded care. Therefore, information on costs and entitlement to treatment is made readily available to patients and prospective patients.

Availability of NHS care

As discussed in Chapter 41, dentists are independent contractors and can contract to provide as much or as little NHS care as they wish. Prior to 2006, NHS dental care was funded by a non-cash-limited budget and health authorities were obliged to contract with appropriately qualified and registered dentists. This is no longer the case, and indeed, dentists can only opt to provide NHS care if they can negotiate a contract with NHS England or their local Health Board in Wales and Scotland and the equivalent Board in Northern Ireland.

The backlog in dental care caused by the COVID-19 pandemic and unhappiness with the terms of the NHS contract on the part of providing dentists and dental care professionals has resulted in an acute crisis in access to dental care in many parts of the United Kingdom. This has received much attention in the media. A survey conducted by the British Broadcasting Corporation (BBC) in August 2022 claimed that 9 in 10 NHS dental practices across the UK were not accepting new adult patients for treatment under the health service. Terms such as 'dental deserts', used to describe areas where there are no NHS dental providers or no providers willing to take on new patients, have become common parlance.

Rural and remote communities

Access to dental care can be a problem in rural and remote communities. In addition to access to NHS dental services, issues such as distance to travel, lack of adequate public transport facilities and unwillingness of young practitioners to work in rural and remote areas all contribute to the problem.

Access to care for patients with disabilities

Patients with mental and physical disabilities may experience difficulty in accessing care (Chapter 36).

Barriers interact in complex ways

Often, issues over adequate access to dental care are not due to one single barrier but to a combination of factors that interact in complex ways and to greater or lesser degrees in any given patient (Figure 42.2).

43 Migration, race and ethnicity

Figure 43.1 The stages on a migrant's journey

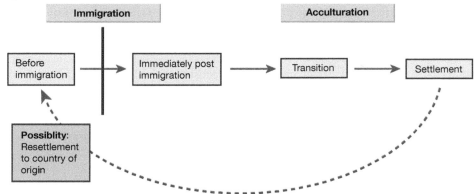

Table 43.1 Beliefs, traditions and cultural issues that may have impacts on dental care

Differences in habits, customs, beliefs, practices and other factors can have impacts on oral health-related behaviours and on the uptake and delivery of dental care. The following are issues with which members of the dental team should be familiar.

Factor	Issue	Examples
Health beliefs and understanding of disease	Different cultures have different health beliefs	Chinese people believe in the concept of yin and yang. This may influence their dietary choices, foods being balanced between yin (cold) and yang (hot). Remedies from traditional Chinese medicine may form part of their management of oral problems.
Gender issues and ideas of modesty	A religious protocol may dictate preferences when undergoing dental care	Modesty is important in all aspects of Muslim life, extending to healthcare. Muslim women may prefer to be treated by female dentists.
Dietary restrictions	Avoidance of certain foods is important in many religions	Neither Jews nor Muslims eat pork. Certain dental materials, e.g. collagen sutures and periodontal chips, are porcine in origin. Patients should be made aware of this, and an alternative should be agreed.
	Avoidance of alcohol is common in many religions	Strict observance will want to use an alcohol-free mouthwash. On occasion, questions arise as to whether fluoride varnish is appropriate for the children of faiths that avoid alcohol (alcohol, present in trace amounts, acts as a solvent in fluoride varnish). Guidance from religious leaders suggests that this is not an issue. The alcohol is not consumed for pleasure and is not swallowed.
Fasting	Fasting is a common religious practice	During the holy month of Ramadan, Muslims fast from sun up to sun-down. Patients may wish to avoid non-urgent dental treatment during this period and appointments should be scheduled accordingly.
Oral hygiene practices different approaches to dental treatment	Non-Western techniques of tooth cleaning may be preferred Approaches to dental treatment vary in different parts of the world	Some patients, particularly older patients of Middle Eastern or African origin, may prefer to clean their teeth with a miswak – a fibrous root-though this is observed much less commonly than previously. Dentistry in Eastern Europe (former Soviet bloc countries) often takes the form of 'heavy-duty' multiple fixed prostheses.
Tooth modification	Body modification and adornment have existed since the earliest times	Modification of the form and function of dentition is still practised in many parts of the world and may be encountered when providing dental care. 'Dental grillz'/ gold crowns in rappers are one current form of tooth adornment.
Language	Language-related issues	See Table 43.2.
Health literacy	Health literacy describes the ability to understand information related to health improvement and healthcare	Connected closely to language issues, unfamiliarity with Western dental care and practices can hinder understanding.
Torture	Asylum seekers may have been mistreated	Previous mistreatment involving the head and mouth as a form of punishment or torture should be borne in mind if treating a patient who has sought asylum.
Consent	For consent to treatment to be valid it needs to be informed	Where a dentist and patient do not share a common language, ensuring that the patient fully understands and agrees with the proposed treatment can be a problem.

Dental Public Health at a Glance, Second Edition. Ivor G. Chestnutt.
© 2024 John Wiley & Sons Ltd. Published 2024 by John Wiley & Sons Ltd.

The United Kingdom as a multicultural society

The 2021 Census showed that one in six usual residents of England and Wales were born outside the UK, an increase of 2.5 million since 2011, from 7.5 million (13.4%) to 10 million (16.8%). India remained the most common country of birth outside the UK in 2021 (920,000 people, 1.5% of all usual residents). The number of people who were born in Romania and are now resident in the UK grew by 576% since the previous census, from 80,000 in 2011 to 539,000 in 2021. These data emphasise the multicultural nature of British society. This has implications for the organisation and delivery of dental care.

Migration

A migrant is defined by the United Nations as:

a person who moves to a country other than that of his or her usual residence for a period of at least a year.

A number of different categories of migrants can be identified: migrant workers, students, asylum seekers and refugees, victims of trafficking and reunified family members.

Race and ethnicity

It is important to understand the difference between race and ethnicity.
• Race is one of the major subdivisions of humankind, based largely on phenotypical differences between peoples.
• Ethnicity is a social construct that is based on common national or cultural traditions.

There is very limited evidence that racial characteristics have a great impact on susceptibility to dental diseases. Some studies have suggested that some racial groups may be more susceptible to aggressive forms of periodontitis.

Of much greater significance is the impact of ethnic and cultural factors. Differences in habits, customs, beliefs and practices can have significant impacts on susceptibility to oral disease and to the uptake and acceptability of dental care in a number of ways (Table 43.1).

Ethnicity and social and economic deprivation

The impact of social and economic factors on health is discussed in Chapter 19. It should always be remembered that minority communities frequently live in disadvantaged circumstances. In determining the impact of ethnic and cultural practices, the confounding effect of poverty needs to be carefully disentangled. Thus, for example, do the higher rates of dental caries observed in minority ethnic children in England reflect underlying cultural practices, or is caries prevalence in these children no different from that in impoverished white children? Research studies are conflicting on the answer to this question.

Migration and health

Migrants' health can be influenced by factors at play during different stages of the immigration cycle (Figure 43.1). Typically, newly arrived immigrants are young and relatively healthy, but as they adapt to the lifestyle and practices in their adopted country (i.e. become acculturated), they more and more experience similar diseases to the indigenous population. Migrants tend to be more vulnerable to diabetes, certain communicable diseases, maternal and child health problems, occupational health hazards and poor mental health. Obesity is increasingly recognised as a problem when migrants move from a low-income country to a developed country.

Access to healthcare

Access to healthcare can be a particular problem for migrants. Language issues are often a barrier; steps to overcome these are shown in Table 43.2. General health literacy, social exclusion and discrimination (both obvious and concealed) are further barriers.

Irregular (illegal) immigrants who do not comply with entry, exit, visa and work permit requirements are particularly likely to experience difficulty in accessing health services.

Migrant clinicians and health workers

The National Health Service has for many years relied on healthcare professionals trained overseas to meet its workforce requirements. In addition, a growing number of dependent elderly people in nursing and care homes often rely on low-skilled migrant workers to provide basic care.

Overseas trained dentists

Dentists who have qualified at a dental school in the European Union are entitled to work in the United Kingdom (UK) under freedom of movement regulations. The European Directive on the Recognition of Professional Qualifications for Dentists enables European Economic Area (EEA) nationals who qualified at a dental school in the EEA to practise anywhere in the EEA without the need to undertake further education or training. To date, this has not been significantly affected by the UK's decision to leave the European Union. The UK government enacted legislation that enabled the General Dental Council (GDC) to continue recognising EEA-qualified dentists under a near-automatic system. These arrangements were reviewed by the UK Government in the first half of 2023 and extended for a period of five years.

Dentists who are qualified elsewhere in the world who wish to practice in the UK have to sit and pass the Overseas Registration Examination administered by the GDC. There have been lengthy waits to gain a place to sit this examination and the GDC is, at the time of writing, undertaking a consultation on the arrangements for admitting overseas qualified dental professionals to the Register. Those qualified outside the UK should consult the GDC website to understand arrangements.

Differences in competencies acquired during undergraduate training and unfamiliarity with NHS Dental Regulations are potential problems for dentists coming to work in the United Kingdom. NHS Commissioners have been proactive in organising additional skills training for practitioners in this position.

Cultural competence

In an increasingly diverse society, it is important that both healthcare organisations and healthcare professionals are culturally competent. This means that they need to be aware of the types of issues addressed in this chapter.

Table 43.2 Options to manage an encounter when clinician and patient do not share a common language

Method of translation	Notes
Face-to-face translation by a friend or relative	The most common, but least satisfactory method; can be difficult to ensure that the dentist is hearing the patient's view and not the relative's view
Face-to-face translation by a professional translator	The preferred option; not always available; expensive; needs arranging in advance; may not be available in an emergency situation
Use of a professional telephone translation service	Lacks the face-to-face element – difficult when undertaking treatment
Use of bilingual cards and photographs	It can be of some help, particularly if the parties share a little of a common language – it is not possible to have to hand all of the many languages that could possibly be encountered

Skill mix in dentistry

Table 44.1 Total number of people on the Dentists Register and the Dental Care Professionals Register at the end of 2022 by gender

		Male	Female
Dentist	44.125	21,179 (48.0%)	22,946 (52.0%)
Dental care professional (DCP)	71,326	5160 (7.2%)	66,166 (92.8%)
Total	**115,451**	**26,339 (22.1%)**	**89,112 (77.2%)**

Source: *Data from General Dental Council (2022).*

Table 44.2 The composition of the United Kingdom General Dental Council Register by professional group, December 2022

Registration title	Number of dental professionals	Percentage of professionals on the register
Clinical Dental Technician	395	<1%
Dentist	44,125	36%
Dental Hygienist	8699	7%
Dental Nurse	58,292	47.5%
Dental Technician	5107	4%
Dental Therapist	4916	4%
Orthodontic Therapist	898	1%
Total	**122,432**	**100%**

Totals do not match those in Table 44.1 as individuals may be registered in more than one category of professional.
Source: *General Dental Council, Registration Statistical Report (2022).*

Table 44.3 Scope of practice of dental therapists in the UK

Dental therapists are registered dental professionals who provide certain items of dental treatment directly to patients or under prescription from a dentist.

If trained, competent and appropriately indemnified, dental therapists can:
- Obtain a detailed dental history from patients and evaluate their medical history.
- Carry out a clinical examination within their competence.
- Complete periodontal examination and charting and use indices to screen and monitor periodontal disease.
- Diagnose and devise a treatment plan within their competence.
- Prescribe radiographs.
- Take, process and interpret various film views used in general dental practice.
- Plan the delivery of care for patients.
- Give appropriate patient advice.
- Provide preventive oral care to patients and liaise with dentists to treat caries, periodontal disease and tooth wear.
- Undertake supragingival and subgingival scaling and root surface debridement using manual and powered instruments.
- Use appropriate antimicrobial therapy to manage plaque-related diseases.
- Adjust restored surfaces in relation to periodontal treatment.
- Apply topical treatments and fissure sealants.
- Give patients advice on how to stop smoking.
- Take intra- and extraoral photographs.
- Give infiltration and inferior dental block analgesia.
- Place temporary dressings and re-cement crowns with temporary cement.
- Place rubber dam.
- Take impressions.
- Take care of implants and provide treatment for peri-implant tissues.
- Carry out direct restorations on primary and secondary teeth.
- Carry out pulpotomies on primary teeth.
- Extract primary teeth.
- Place pre-formed crowns on primary teeth.
- Identify anatomical features, recognise abnormalities and interpret common pathology.
- Carry out oral cancer screening.
- If necessary, refer patients to other healthcare professionals.
- Keep full, accurate and contemporaneous patient records.
- If working on a prescription, vary the detail but not the direction of the prescription according to patient needs. For example, the number of surfaces to be restored or other materials to be used.

Additional skills that dental therapists could develop include:
- Carrying out tooth whitening to the prescription of a dentist.
- Administering inhalation sedation.
- Removing sutures after the wound has been checked by a dentist. All other skills are reserved to orthodontic therapists, dental technicians, clinical dental technicians or dentists.

Source: *Data from General Dental Council (2013).*

The concept of skill mix

The tasks required to provide comprehensive healthcare are not of equal complexity. As both the number of staff and the amount of finance in any healthcare system are finite, the delivery of healthcare can be made more efficient by the use of a mix of staff trained to various levels. This allows the most highly trained staff to delegate aspects of care to other professionals. This concept is known as skill mix. It has been widely adopted in medicine, and many procedures that would previously have been conducted by a medical practitioner are now delegated to a nurse. The skill mix in dentistry currently lags behind that in medicine.

Skill mix in dentistry

The idea of dental care professionals (previously termed auxiliaries) has existed for 100 years, and in 1916, the School Dental Service in the United Kingdom employed dental dressers (the equivalent of dental therapists). These workers were phased out in the early 1920s following the passing of the Dentists Act 1921. The first dental hygienists in the United Kingdom were trained by the military in 1943, with civilian schools of dental hygiene being established in the 1950s. Training of dental therapists began formally in the 1960s in London. Until the early 2000s, dental therapists were restricted to working in Hospital and Community Dental Services, but changed legislation means that dental therapists can now work in general dental practice.

The concept of dental care, delivered by a multi-skilled team, was given prominence by a report from the Nuffield Foundation in 1993 and subsequently endorsed by a General Dental Council (GDC) sponsored review of the use of dental auxiliaries in 1998. The model of a primary care dental team, led by a dentist who diagnoses, prescribes and delegates routine clinical care to a team of support professionals (dental nurses, hygienists, therapists and technicians), is now accepted in the United Kingdom.

All dentists and dental care professionals (DCPs) are required to register with the GDC. The number of individuals registered. The number of DCPs and categories of professionals recognised by the GDC are shown in Tables 44.1 and 44.2, respectively.

In the past two decades, the range of tasks that DCPs can train to undertake has expanded markedly. In 2013, the GDC granted direct access to some categories of DCP. This means that patients can see dental hygienists and therapists without first having to see a dentist or without the need for a prescription. The degree to which this has proven possible in the period since then has been limited. The potential impact of direct access to DCPS on the delivery of dental care has still to be established.

Tasks that can be undertaken by dental care professionals

The list of competencies expected of all dental professionals is set out in guidance from the GDC entitled Preparing for Practice–Dental Team Learning, Outcomes for Registration (www.gdc-uk.org). This list of competencies was last revised in 2015. Like dentists, the proficiencies required of DCPs are described in four domains:
- Clinical
- Communication
- Professionalism
- Management and leadership.

The scope of practice of individual registrant groups is also defined by the GDC. It sets out the areas of dental practice that a given professional group could be expected and trained to perform. These are set out in detail for dentists and for each DCP group in a GDC publication, Scope of Practice 2013. The scope of practice for dental therapists is shown in Table 44.3. The GDC regularly reviews the learning outcomes associated with dental education courses, and such a review is currently underway.

Dentists should be aware of the range of skills and duties that fall within the remit of each DCP group and delegate care accordingly. Like dentists, DCPs have a duty to undertake life-long learning and to make an annual return to the GDC to enable their ongoing registration (Chapter 48). It is expected that DCPs will have the opportunity to develop and enhance their skills in the course of a career in practice.

Skill mix – an international perspective

Dental therapists

The first formal training programme for dental therapists was established in New Zealand in 1923 with two further schools opened in the 1950s. It was largely the success of the New Zealand model that encouraged the establishment of a training programme in London in the 1960s. Despite the long history of dental therapists treating children in New Zealand and the United Kingdom, the concept of dental therapists has not been widely adopted around the world. Often, vested interests and the strength of national dental associations have been set against the development of this class of dental professionals. At present, vigorous debate continues in the United States as to the merits of employing dental therapists despite many thousands of uninsured high-need children in that country who do not have access to routine dental care.

Dental hygienists

Dental hygienists, with their more restricted remit, have seen much wider acceptance by the dental profession across the world. Dental hygienists are widely employed in Scandinavian countries and in the United States. However, they are much less common in southern European countries and are not used in Austria, Belgium, France, Greece or Luxembourg.

Dental nurses

While the concept of four-handed dentistry is firmly established in the United Kingdom and many other countries, the use of dental nurses or dental assistants is not universal. Direct chairside assistants are relatively uncommon in Luxembourg and France.

Clinical dental technicians

As well as being registered in the United Kingdom, clinical dental technicians are found in Denmark and France, where they can provide removable dental prostheses directly to patients.

45 Pandemics and other threats in the context of providing dental services

Figure 45.1 Number of adults and children accessing general dental services in England, January 2019 to October 2020. Source: *The impact of the COVID-19 pandemic on oral health inequalities and access to oral healthcare in England | British Dental Journal (nature.com).*

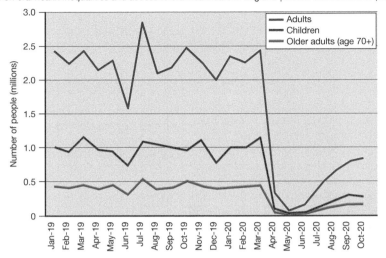

Figure 45.2 Impacts of the COVID-19 pandemic on dentistry

Only urgent dental care was possible in the initial stages of the pandemic	Reduced patient flow whist 'fallow time' was observed between patients to allow aerosols to settle
Disruption to dental education and training	Costs of increased 'personal protective equipment (PPE)'
Disruption caused by Long-Covid affecting both patients and staff	
The mental health of dental care professionals deteriorated	Finances of purchasing air purifying equipment / air extraction systems
Backlog of patients needing care resulted in long waiting lists-especially for specialist procedures requiring hospital admission	Disruption to the financial model on which many dental practices (especially NHS practices) operated
Progression of dental disease due to delayed appointments	Patients delayed care due to fear of catching the virus

The COVID-19 pandemic

The COVID-19 pandemic resulted from a global outbreak of coronavirus, an infectious disease caused by the severe acute respiratory syndrome coronavirus 2 (SARS-CoV-2) virus. The virus is thought to have been transmitted from an animal source, most likely originating in a bat. The first cases of novel coronavirus (nCoV) were detected in China in December 2019, with the virus spreading rapidly to other countries across the world. This led the World Health Organisation (WHO) to declare a Public Health Emergency of International Concern (PHEIC) on 30 January 2020 and to characterise the outbreak as a pandemic on 11 March 2020.

By May 2023, the WHO said that given the disease was by now well-established and ongoing, it no longer fitted the definition of a PHEIC. This did not mean the pandemic itself was over, but the global emergency had ended, for now.

Definition of a pandemic

A pandemic is an outbreak of infectious disease that occurs over a wide geographical area and that is of high prevalence. A pandemic generally affects a significant proportion of the world's population, usually over the course of several months.

Impact of the COVID-19 pandemic

Impact in general

The COVID-19 pandemic has been the single greatest disruptor of life in the twenty-first century. The WHO reported that by September 2023, globally, there had been 770,563,467 confirmed cases of COVID-19, including 6,957,216 deaths. The corresponding figures for the United Kingdom were 24,704,113 cases and 229,389 deaths. These data are likely to underestimate the full impact of the virus.

Dental Public Health at a Glance, Second Edition. Ivor G. Chestnutt.
© 2024 John Wiley & Sons Ltd. Published 2024 by John Wiley & Sons Ltd.

In the immediate aftermath of the declaration of the pandemic, governments in many countries took drastic action to prevent the spread of the virus. In the UK, for a time, only essential workers were permitted to leave their homes (other than to exercise or buy essential food items) as the most severe restrictions on civil activities for generations were imposed. International travel was severely curtailed.

Impact on healthcare systems

Health systems were put under enormous strain as they tried to cope with the unprecedented influx of patients, many of whom required intensive support. Healthcare professionals were under massive pressure as they worked out the most appropriate regimen for treating this new disease, which, although primarily a respiratory virus, impacted multiple body systems.

The life-preserving breakthrough came when, in December 2020 the UK authorities became the first to approve the use of a vaccine against the SARS-CoV-2 virus. This happened because of unprecedented cooperation between researchers, pharmaceutical companies, governments and the regulatory authorities. Mass vaccination programmes were implemented and have contained the virus. However, the SARS-CoV-2 virus remains a dangerous pathogen and continual vigilance on the part of public health authorities is required to identify outbreaks, particularly those which result from a new variant of the virus.

As health systems dealt with the victims of the SARS-CoV-2 virus, routine care was suspended for all but the most life-threatening conditions. This resulted in a significant backlog of patients awaiting treatment. In September 2023, NHS England's waiting list for treatment stood at 7.7 million people, an all-time record.

The COVID-19 pandemic and dentistry

The pandemic had significant implications for dental professionals, dental care and oral health improvement programmes. The immediate impact of the 'stay at home' restrictions imposed in the UK on the delivery of dental care is shown in Figures 45.1 and 45.2. For a period, only emergency dental care was available.

As a respiratory virus transmitted primarily via droplet spread, SARS-CoV-2 virus posed problems for the delivery of dental care, particularly for those procedures that involved the generation of aerosols (e.g. use of high-speed drills, ultra-sonic scalers). The need to introduce 'fallow-time' – that is a period between patients when a clinic was left empty to allow aerosols to settle, significantly reducing the capacity and throughput of patients.

Issues impacting dentistry are summarised in Figure 45.1.

The disruption caused by COVID-19 significantly impacted on the financial stability of many dental practices, although NHS commissioners were largely sympathetic by relaxing expectations in terms of service delivery.

The suspension of schools and the introduction of at-home learning meant that in-school oral health improvement programmes such as Designed to Smile in Wales and Childsmile in Scotland had to cease. Many of the staff employed by the NHS to deliver such programmes were redeployed to work in mass vaccination centres.

Other infectious diseases that have impacted on the delivery of dental care

At the commencement of the COVID-19 pandemic, dentistry was advantaged by the already high standards of infection prevention and control that were in place. In contrast with many other healthcare providers, dental staff routinely wore masks, eye protection and gloves when undertaking clinical procedures. This reflects the long-standing awareness of the heavily contaminated environment that comprises the oral cavity. It is not unprecedented for a newly emerged pathogen to impact on how dental care is delivered. Significant changes were seen after the emergence of the Human Immunodeficiency Virus (HIV) and the prion induced, Bovine Spongiform Encephalitis (Box 45.1).

Surveillance role of public health

Public health practitioners were central in providing advice to governments and other authorities in the course of the recent pandemic. It is the role of public health to continually survey and scan for the next potentially lethal infectious agent to emerge. Knowing which new agent will have the devastating impact on humanity that has been seen with the SARS-CoV-2 virus is difficult.

In the UK, the government has been subject to criticism over just how prepared the nation was for a pandemic, for the mechanisms employed to procure personal protective equipment and a belief that the next pandemic would arise from an influenza virus.

Without a doubt the ability to produce an effective vaccination and to have this made available to the populus within 12 months of the virus emerging was key to averting an even greater disaster afflicting humanity.

Box 45.1 Changes in the delivery of Dental Care following the emergence of (a) Human Immunodeficiency Virus and (b) Bovine Spongiform Encephalopathy

Human Immunodeficiency Virus (HIV)

The emergence of the Human Immunodeficiency Virus in the early 1980s led to the routine wearing of clinical gloves by dental professionals. When the virus first emerged, for a time, extreme measures were taken when treating patients known to be infected with HIV. However, more proportionate measures were adopted in due course.

The issue in taking additional cross-infection control measures when treating patients infected with a newly emerged pathogen is: 'What about patients who are unknowingly infected with the pathogen, those in the pre-symptomatic phase or who are asymptomatic?'

For that reason, the most sensible approach is to adopt 'universal infection control measures'. That means all patients should be regarded as 'infectious' or 'potentially infectious'. In that way, everyone is protected. This approach has the added advantage of not stigmatising patients.

Nonetheless, there are circumstances in the wider healthcare arena where patients infected with highly infectious pathogens will need to be 'barrier nursed' in specialist units. Clearly, dental care for such patients would be delayed until they have recovered/are no longer infectious.

Bovine spongiform encephalopathy (BSE)

Bovine spongiform encephalopathy, commonly known as mad cow disease, is an incurable and invariably fatal neurodegenerative disease of cattle. Spread to humans is believed to result in variant Creutzfeldt–Jakob disease (vCJD). As of 2018, a total of 231 cases of vCJD had been reported globally. The disease is thought to have been caused by feeding infected animal products to animals. In the early-mid 1990s, there was great concern that a pandemic of individuals infected with vCJD was possible and about four million cows were slaughtered and disposed of in the UK during the eradication process. The disease is caused by a prion - a misfolded protein.

Concerns that this protein might be harboured in human neurological tissue, including the dental pulp, resulted in the introduction of more stringent cross-infection control procedures such as: greater use of single-use instruments, increased disinfection and autoclaving requirements for used surgical instruments; traceability of used instruments following surgery.

46 The environmental agenda and dentistry

Figure 46.1   The pathways by which climate change can impact on health. Source: *Adapted from WHO: Climate Change and health (2023).*

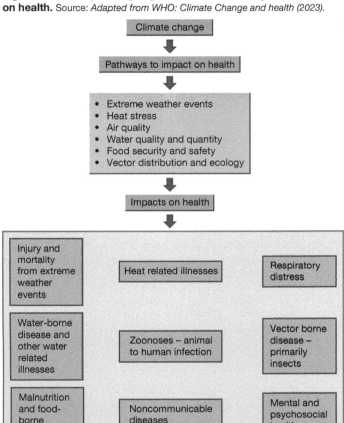

Figure 46.2   The Total annual carbon footprint of dental services in England – 2013/2014. Source: *Reproduced from Carbon Modelling Within Dentistry / Crown / Licensed under CC BY 3.0.*

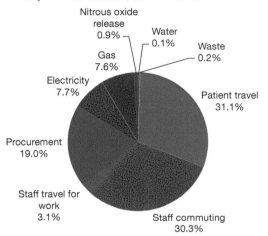

Nitrous oxide release 0.9%
Water 0.1%
Gas 7.6%
Waste 0.2%
Electricity 7.7%
Patient travel 31.1%
Procurement 19.0%
Staff travel for work 3.1%
Staff commuting 30.3%

Table 46.1 The contribution of different dental procedures to the overall carbon footprint of NHS dental care in England, 2013–2014

Dental procedure	Contribution to total carbon footprint from NHS dentistry (%)
Dental examination	27.1
Scale and polish	13.4
Amalgam fillings	9.7
Composite fillings	9.5
Acrylic dentures	8.6
Radiographs	6.4
Extraction of teeth	3.5
Non-precious metal crowns	3.3
Fluoride varnish	2.9
Endodontic treatment	2.1
Study models	1.6
Glass ionomer fillings	1.5
Precious metal crowns, metal dentures, fissure sealants, porcelain crowns	Each < 1%

Sources: *Public Health England/Centre for Sustainable Health Care (2018).*

The impact of climate change on health

The World Health Organisation (WHO) has said that changes to the climate are the single greatest threat to humanity. Between 2030 and 2050, climate change is expected to cause approximately 250,000 additional deaths per year, from malnutrition, malaria, diarrhoea and heat stress.

The impact of global warming on health and healthcare has a number of dimensions. The greatest is the effect on the social and environmental determinants of health – clean air, safe drinking water, sufficient food and secure shelter (Figure 46.1). These are likely to have the greatest impact on low-income and developing countries who have the least ability to cope with the changes envisaged. This has the potential to widen global health inequalities.

Effects are also apparent in developed countries. Maximum temperature records were broken in the United Kingdom in the summer of 2022. In some locations, the temperature exceeded 40°C for the

Dental Public Health at a Glance, Second Edition. Ivor G. Chestnutt.
© 2024 John Wiley & Sons Ltd. Published 2024 by John Wiley & Sons Ltd.

first time. During the five heat periods between June and August 2022 (defined as day(s) on which a Level 3 Heat Health Alert is issued and/or day(s) when the mean Central England Temperature is greater than 20°C), 56,303 deaths occurred in England and Wales. According to the Office for National Statistics, that was 3,271 deaths (6.2%) above the five-year average. Between 10 and 25 July 2022, there were 2227 excess deaths – 10.4% above average.

The impact of climate change on healthcare

Clearly, if unaddressed, the increased morbidity and mortality associated with climate change will have significant implications for healthcare and climate-resilient facilities, which need to be planned for.

It is also important to review what hospitals and clinics can do to make their contribution to a more environmentally friendly environment. Hospitals emit large amounts of greenhouse gases in their healthcare delivery through transportation, waste and other resources and are considered as key players in reducing healthcare's environmental footprint. Most areas of healthcare are working to achieve environmentally sustainable practices. There are implications for dental care.

Sustainable dental care

An analysis by Public Health England from 2013 to 2014 estimated the total greenhouse gas emissions of NHS dental services in England measured in tonnes of carbon dioxide equivalents (tCO2e) was 675,706. That is the equivalent to flying 50,000 times from the UK to Hong Kong and making up 3% of the overall carbon footprint of the NHS in England. The highest proportion of these emissions was caused by travel, followed by procurement, energy, nitrous oxide, waste and water (Figure 46.2). The relative contribution of different dental procedures to the overall dental carbon footprint is shown in Table 46.1.

Contributors to the carbon footprint in providing dental care and potential mitigating actions

Travel

The greatest impact on the environment as a result of dental care comes from travel to the dental surgery – both staff and patients. Sustainable travel, which encourages walking, cycling and the use of public transport, may benefit patients in attending a dental surgery. This is more likely in an urban than a rural setting where many patients are likely to be reliant on travel by car to their dental appointments.

Commissioners of dental services should bear in mind travel to services. New built clinical facilities should adopt environmentally acceptable and sustainable construction and running facilities such as green power, building insulation, solar panelling, alternative lighting and heating and other energy-intensive aspects of operating the building.

Single-use equipment

The trend towards single-use equipment and prepackaged/pre-sterilised equipment has the potential to result in a greater impact on the environment. A balance needs to be struck between maximising infection prevention and control, the convenience of use and environmental impact.

Waste disposal

Dental surgeries generate considerable volumes of waste, both domestic and clinical. Regulations must be complied with in relation to the disposal of infected waste, but whenever possible, waste recycling should be adopted. Waste reduction can be achieved through more effective stock management, recycling or replacing disposable plastic materials with reusable alternatives.

Radiography chemicals

Conventional radiography generates chemical waste in the form of used processing chemicals like silver and lead. The move to digital radiography has reduced this source of waste.

Dental amalgam

Concerns over the effects of mercury as an environmental contaminant have led to the banning of amalgam in some countries. In the United Kingdom, its use is prohibited in certain patient groups. Separators in chairs are a means of ensuring that waste amalgam does not escape to the wastewater system. The major concern with amalgam is not primarily during the provision of dental care, but rather its escape to the environment postmortem.

Oral hygiene products

Used dental hygiene aids such as toothbrushes, interdental brushes and floss contribute significantly to landfill. Eco-friendly toothbrushes have been marketed, but cost, availability, ease of use and effective plaque removal are all issues with these alternatives. Toothbrush recycling schemes have been facilitated by some commercial companies.

Personal protective equipment

The increased use of personal protective equipment as a result of the COVID-19 pandemic is a further source of potentially contaminated waste.

Digital solutions

Computer use, economical printing and online oral health care management systems can reduce paper waste. The degree to which online consultations are of use in dentistry is uncertain and is likely limited to some specialist settings.

Oral health improvement and climate change

The ultimate goal of dental public health is to prevent oral disease. Prevention of oral disease reduces the need for dental care, thereby reducing the overall impact of dental activity on the environment.

Indirect health benefits of addressing climate change

Transportation produces around 20% of global carbon emissions. Alternatives like walking and cycling are not only green but also offer major health benefits, such as reducing the risk of many chronic health conditions and improving mental health.

47 The future delivery of dental care

Table 47.1 The principles that NHS England wants to apply to reform how General Dental Services are commissioned, 2022

Principles
- Be designed with the support of the profession
- Improve oral health outcomes
- Increase incentives to undertake preventative dentistry, prioritise evidence-based care for patients with the most needs and reduce incentives to deliver care that is of low clinical value
- Improve patient access to NHS care, with a specific focus on addressing inequalities, particularly deprivation and ethnicity
- Demonstrate that patients do not have to pay privately for dental care that was previously commissioned under NHS dental care
- Be affordable within NHS resources made available by Government, including taking account of dental charge income (i.e. patient co-payments).

Table 47.2 Amendments to the General Dental Service Contract in England, July 2022

Amendments
- Introduce enhanced UDAs to support higher-needs patients, recognising the range of different treatment options currently remunerated under Band 2
- Improve monitoring of and adherence to personalised recall intervals
- Establish a new minimum indicative UDA value
- Address misunderstandings around the use of skill mix in NHS dental care whilst removing some of the administrative barriers preventing dental care professionals from operating within their full scope of practice
- Take steps to maximise access from existing NHS resources, including through funding practices to deliver more activity in the year when affordable
- Improve information for patients by requiring more regular updating of the Directory of Services

Table 47.3 Factors impacting the future delivery of dental care

Factors impacting the future delivery of dental care
- Increasing population (absolute numbers)
- Ageing population
- Increased tooth retention into old age
- Changed attitudes to oral health
- The public is less willing to accept extractions
- Ever-rising expectations for good dental appearance
- Need to address inequalities in oral health
- Ever-improving dental technology, which means teeth can be restored that previously would have been extracted
- Advances in restorative dental materials
- Increased demand for cosmetic dental care
- Limited resources to fund NHS dentistry
- Difficulty in workforce planning (Table 47.4)
- Global mobility and European employment legislation have resulted in a much greater number of overseas dentists working in the United Kingdom, but this has been impacted by the United Kingdom's decision to leave the European Union (Brexit)
- The enactment of direct access powers for dental hygienists and therapists means that greater use of skill mix is more likely than has previously been the case
- Geopolitical events like Russia's illegal invasion of Ukraine have impacted the cost of living and monies available to pay for dental care
- Need for dental surgeries to adopt environmentally friendly practices

Table 47.4 Factors in workforce planning

Influencing factors
- The number of dental professionals trained in the UK each year
- The balance between the numbers of dentists and other members of the dental team
- Whether practitioners want to work full-time or part-time
- The number of overseas-trained dentists who want to come and work in the UK and are able to meet the requirements to register with the General Dental Council
- Geopolitical issues like Brexit influence where overseas-trained dentists want to work
- The degree to which UK-trained staff want to work abroad
- The number of current members of the dental team who will retire in the coming years
- Whither dentists will choose to contract with the NHS or wish to provide care privately
- The nature of work dentists want to do
- Whether dental staff are prepared to work in rural and remote areas

National Health Service (NHS dentistry) 1948 to present

When the NHS was established in 1948, oral health in the United Kingdom was extremely poor. However, universal access to dentistry generated by the NHS in the mid-twentieth century meant that patients could be relieved of grossly decayed teeth and provided with complete or partial dentures, which adequately restored form and function, met patients' needs and were a vast improvement in standards at the time. Such was the demand for dental care that in 1952, the concept of dental care free for all at the point of delivery was abandoned, as it became obvious that the State could not afford to pay for all of the dental care the public wished to consume. Means-tested patient charges (co-payments)

Dental Public Health at a Glance, Second Edition. Ivor G. Chestnutt.
© 2024 John Wiley & Sons Ltd. Published 2024 by John Wiley & Sons Ltd.

were introduced. For the remainder of the twentieth century, under a fee-per-item method of payment, the efforts of NHS dentists did much to improve the oral health of the nation (Chapter 9).

Since the 1960s, various reviews and investigations into NHS dentistry have changed how dentists are remunerated. Many of these changes were designed to address the pros and cons of remunerating dentists using fee-per-item versus capitation (Chapter 41). The most significant changes occurred in 1990 and 2006. The last major change in England and Wales happened in 2006 and introduced the concept of Units of Dental Activity and payment bands. For the first time, it also put a limit on the total money available for NHS dentistry each year.

Units of dental activity

This concept was introduced in England and Wales as a contracting currency and was used to replace the traditional fee-per-item method of remunerating dentists for the care that they provide.

Within a short period of time, it was recognised that the 2006 contract reforms were failing to meet the desired objectives – simplifying the payment system and increasing access to NHS dentistry. The main issue was that the transition from a fee-per-item system with over 400 items to a system with effectively three items was not working. There was no incentive to see high-needs patients – greatest rewards came from seeing low-need / low-risk patients at intervals more frequently than was clinically necessary.

The Department of Health in England commissioned an independent review of NHS dentistry in 2009. The model proposed in that review suggested a care pathway in which a patient's oral health and risk of future disease are assessed. The focus of care should be on prevention, tailored to the patient's individual needs. Advanced aspects of care would only be provided when there is a stable oral environment, the patient's disease risks are under control, and the patient is in a continuing care relationship with the dentist/dental team.

The emphasis of the proposed changes was to provide:

NHS dental care refocused from a service designed to provide restorative care to one that is focused on prevention.

Reform of the NHS dental contract

England

For more than a decade, the NHS in both England and Wales have piloted alternative models of commissioning NHS General Dental Services in an attempt to achieve the objectives of the 2009 review. They have, however, been unable to arrive at a definitive and secure model for commissioning dental care. Issues have included an inability to derive a rapid risk assessment tool in England.

The current objectives of the NHS in England in relation to the reform of the General Dental Service Contract are summarised in Table 47.1. NHS England has agreed some modifications to the 2006 contract (Table 47.2), but the struggle to come up with a satisfactory contracting mechanism goes on.

Wales

In Wales, it has been possible to implement a risk assessment tool. Known as an assessment of clinical oral risks and needs (ACORN), this system categorises patients into risk categories (green, amber, red) across three domains (dental caries, periodontal disease and

other dental needs). Units of Dental Activity no longer feature in the revised dental contract in Wales. Instead, practitioners have been set different metrics, including the provision of fluoride varnish, seeing a defined percentage of patients who have not recently attended the practice and seeing urgent patients. It is also no longer possible for patients who have been deemed at low risk (green ACORN scores) to have a dental check-up within the following six months.

Scotland and Northern Ireland

The major reform in 2006 did not apply to Scotland and Northern Ireland. There, the contract is still largely based on a fee-per-item model, but significantly modified from that which existed in the early 2000s.

The future design of NHS dental services

Factors impacting the future delivery of dental care are summarised in Table 47.3.

From the above, it is obvious that designing an NHS dental service that meets the needs of patients, providers and governments has proved a significant challenge. This has been made more difficult as a result of the COVID-19 pandemic and the cost of living crisis resulting from geopolitical events. It is hoped that a service designed to meet the ideals of prevention, care based on need and available to as many people who wish to access the service will be possible. Dentistry is in competition with the many other needs that the NHS has to meet. Ultimately, the funding for the service is a matter for the government and the politicians elected to decide on such matters.

Despite concerns raised in the media over difficulties in access to NHS dental care in many areas in the years immediately following the pandemic, it should be remembered that millions of pounds are available to dentists and their teams to contract to provide state-funded dental care.

Independent dental practice

The independent contractor status of general dental practitioners (Chapter 40) means that dentists can deliver care on a private basis. Given that funds available for providing NHS dental care are finite, people who want to have more advanced forms of care, such as implants or cosmetic dental procedures, will have to seek these outside the NHS. However, the NHS reforms make clear that patients are able to choose such treatments alongside NHS care should they so desire.

Workforce

Having sufficient numbers of dentists and dental care professionals to serve the population is very important. However, forecasting the number required is difficult. Factors influencing workforce availability are shown in Table 47.4. NHS England has produced a long-term workforce plan. That proposes expanding dentistry training places in England from 809 in 2022 to 1133 by 2031. Over the same period, an increase in dental hygiene and therapy places from 370 to 475. That will, of course, require significant investment in new training places and staff to train the increased numbers. The degree to which this aspiration will be met remains to be seen.

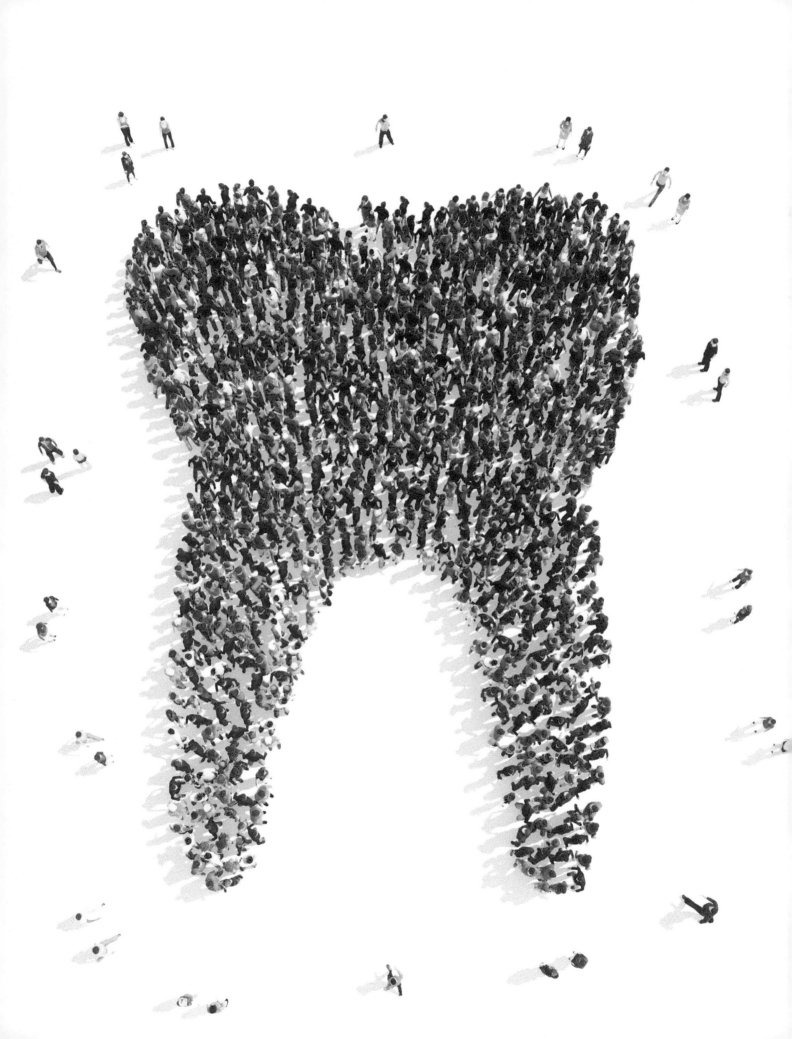

Quality assurance of dental care

Part 11

Chapters

48 Quality dental care

Figure 48.1 The components of quality healthcare

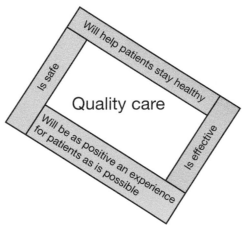

Will help patients stay healthy

Is safe

Quality care

Will be as positive an experience for patients as is possible

Is effective

Table 48.1 Possible consequences of failing to provide quality dental care

A patient may:

- Fail to return for further appointments.
- Tell their family and friends they are dissatisfied with your care and do not recommend your practice. There have been examples of patients posting adverse comments on the internet or social media when dissatisfied with their dental care.
- Complain to the dental practice.
- Complain to the NHS Commissioners, to their insurance provider or the General Dental Council.
- Seek legal redress (sue the dentist or other member of the dental team).

Table 48.3 Examples of risks that need to be managed in dental practice

- Health and safety
  - Slips, trips and falls
  - Cross-infection control
  - Radiation protection
  - Hazardous substances (Committee on Substances Hazardous to Health [COSHH] regulations)
  - Fire evacuation
- Management of medical emergencies
- Patient identification
- Medical records
- Data protection
- Complaints

Table 48.2 Continuing Professional Development requirements determined by the General Dental Council in their Enhanced Scheme (2018)

Requirements

- Complete the minimum number of verifiable CPD hours for your professional title in each five-year cycle.
- Spread CPD across your five-year cycle by completing a minimum of 10 hours of CPD in every two-year period.
- Make a CPD statement as part your annual renewal of registration by making either an annual or end-of-cycle statement, even if you have not completed any CPD during that year.
- Ensure your CPD is relevant to your field(s) of practice.

Recording CPD requirements

- maintaining a personal development plan
- linking activities to at least one development outcome
- keeping a certificate to evidence verifiable CPD.

Hours of CPD required per 5-yr cycle

- dentists need to do a minimum of 100 h
- dental therapists, dental hygienists, orthodontic therapists and clinical dental technicians need to do 75 h
- dental nurses and dental technicians need to do 50 h.

GDC-prescribed Development Outcome categories

A Effective communication with patients, the dental team and others across dentistry, including when obtaining consent, dealing with complaints, and raising concerns when patients are at risk.
B Effective management of self and effective management of others or effective work with others in the dental team, in the interests of patients, providing constructive leadership where appropriate.
C Maintenance and development of your knowledge and skills within your field(s) of practice.
D Maintenance of skills, behaviours and attitudes which maintain patient confidence in your and the dental professions and put patients' interests first.

Dental Public Health at a Glance, Second Edition. Ivor G. Chestnutt.
© 2024 John Wiley & Sons Ltd. Published 2024 by John Wiley & Sons Ltd.

Quality in healthcare

Quality equates to a degree or standard of excellence. Patients quite rightly expect care to be of a certain standard and to maximise their health. There are three components to high-quality care: clinical effectiveness, safety and patient experience (Figure 48.1).

These concepts encompass the six dimensions of healthcare quality defined by Maxell in 1984:

- Access to services
- Relevance to need (for the whole community)
- Effectiveness (for individual patients)
- Equity (fairness)
- Social acceptability
- Efficiency and economy.

In an era when patients increasingly have to pay directly for dental care and when dental practitioners are, in effect, running a business, as in other walks of life, patients expect a quality service. Recent high-profile failures in the provision of healthcare, where serious deficiencies in the commissioning, organisation and delivery of healthcare were ignored, have heightened the focus on providing quality healthcare and ensuring that mechanisms are in place to monitor the provision of care.

The possible consequences of failing to provide quality dental care are shown in Table 48.1.

Clinical governance

Clinical governance is a framework that is designed to ensure that the quality of care patients receive is of a high standard. As the current jargon goes, it is about ensuring that patients get the right care at the right time from the right person and that it happens right the first time. The formal definition of clinical governance is:

A framework through which NHS organisations are accountable for continuously improving the quality of their services and safeguarding high standards of care by creating an environment in which excellence in clinical care will flourish. (Scally and Donaldson 1998)

Clinical governance has the following main components:

1 Clinical audit: See Chapter 49.

2 Clinical effectiveness and evidence-based dentistry: See Chapter 18.

3 Research and development: Healthcare providers are encouraged to participate in research to inform the development of evidence for best practice.

4 Continuing professional development (CPD): It is expected that all healthcare professionals will take steps to keep themselves up to date throughout their practising careers. This is monitored by the General Dental Council (GDC), and all registered dental professionals must make an annual return to confirm that they comply with the minimum expectations. The GDC determines a minimum number of hours that must be committed to CPD over five years and has also identified key topics that should be covered (Table 48.2).

5 Risk management: The practice of dentistry and the dental environment pose risks to patients, staff and visitors. Dental professionals have a duty to manage such risks and to minimise harm to patients by:

- Identifying what can and does go wrong in the delivery of dental care.
- Understanding the factors that influence this.
- Learning lessons from any adverse events.
- Ensuring that action is taken to prevent recurrence.
- Putting systems in place to reduce risk.

The major risks that need to be managed in a dental practice are shown in Table 48.3.

6 Effective management of poorly performing staff: Dentists have a responsibility to ensure that staff working under their supervision are effectively managed and supported. Dental staff may underperform for many reasons, including:

- Professional isolation
- Workload problems
- Lack of continuing professional development (CPD)
- Low morale
- Poor health related to physical or mental problems, alcohol or stress
- Family/other problems outside work.

Dental professionals have an obligation to take action if they suspect that the performance of a colleague or member of staff is such that it may jeopardise the health or welfare of patients or other members of the team. Arrangements should be in place for staff to raise concerns confidentially (whistleblowing, i.e. making a disclosure in the public interest) without fear of retribution.

The 'NHS Patient Safety Strategy' describes how the NHS will continuously improve patient safety, building on the foundations of a safer culture and safer systems.

7 Involvement of patients: It is crucial to a quality dental service that patients' views and wishes are considered. This may be facilitated by the Patient Advice and Liaison Service (PALS), which offers confidential advice and support on healthcare-related matters.

A similar function is fulfilled by Llais in Wales and by the Patient Advice & Support Service in Scotland.

Human factors

Recently, interest has grown in understanding how 'human factors' can impact patient safety in clinical settings, learning from other safety-critical settings such as commercial aviation. Human factor approaches apply knowledge about human behaviour, motives, abilities, limitations and other characteristics to gain a complete understanding of the improved performance of the team. The Human Factors strategies most likely to be effective are those that 'design out' the chance of an error or adverse event occurring.

Excellent communication between team members, effective leadership, civility (that is, treating everyone with politeness and respect) and psychological safety are viewed as key factors in improving patient safety. Psychological safety means being able to speak up and voice concerns without fear of criticism or belittlement.

49 Clinical audit

Figure 49.1 The clinical audit cycle

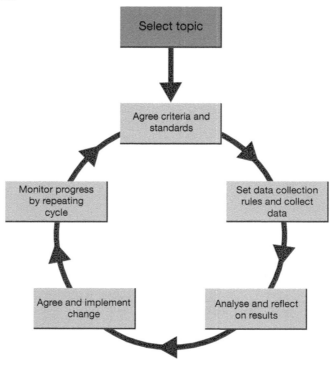

Select topic

Agree criteria and standards

Monitor progress by repeating cycle

Set data collection rules and collect data

Agree and implement change

Analyse and reflect on results

Table 49.1 Reasons for undertaking a clinical audit

- Improved care of patients
- Enhanced professionalism of staff
- Efficient use of resources
- Aid to the administration of dental practice
- Aid to continuing education
- Accountability to those outside the profession
- Requirement of employing organisations and often a condition of employment

Table 49.2 The features of a good clinical audit project

- Effective at improving care
- Not too complicated
- Has a clear purpose
- Assists staff
- Not used as a means of discipline
- Confidential

Table 49.3 Practical issues that may limit the implementation of clinical audit

- Often, audits do not complete the loop due to participant fatigue
- Clinical audit may be seen as a threat or implied criticism
- Viewed as time-consuming
- May choose topics that are not clinically significant
- There is an 'opportunity cost' in doing the audit – time spent on audit activities cannot be spent doing something else

Clinical audit

Clinical audit is central to ensuring that quality dental care is being delivered. Clinical audit can be defined as follows:

Clinical audit is the process of reviewing the delivery of healthcare to identify deficiencies so that they may be remedied.

A clinical audit is a cyclical process in which current care is compared with a standard, and changes are implemented if the standard is not achieved (Figure 49.1). The rationale and benefits of clinical audit are shown in Table 49.1.

The clinical audit cycle

A clinical audit involves the following steps.

1 Deciding on the topic for the audit

The topic chosen for audit should relate to a clinically important aspect of care or a significant event. Subjects for audit may be identified by the observations of staff or arise from patient comments or complaints. Clinical guidelines may also highlight suitable topics for audit.

2 Agree to criteria and standards

A **criterion** is a specific statement of what should be happening.

A **standard** is a minimum level of acceptable performance.

For some topics, criteria and standards are defined by clinical guidelines, for instance, the standards produced by the College of General Dentistry on the quality of radiographs or by the National Institute for Health and Care Excellence (NICE) on the frequency of dental recall intervals. For other topics, there are no national guidelines, and it is up to the team conducting the audit to agree on their own acceptable criteria and standards, as in the following examples:

Criterion	Standard
All patients should have a completed, up-to-date medical history before treatment commences.	Minimum 100%
All patients should be seen within 15 min of their appointment time	Minimum 75%

Here it is clear that the standard for up-to-date medical histories should be 100%, but in the case of keeping patients waiting beyond their appointed treatment time, the standard would be a matter for local decision-making.

3 Data collection

The data required for the audit may already be available from patients' records. Electronic patient record systems have greatly facilitated the retrieval of information on all patients who underwent a particular procedure and avoided the lengthy process of data retrieval from paper-based records.

The information necessary to conduct an audit may need to be collected prospectively via a data collection chart or questionnaire. It is important that the data collection process is kept as simple as possible and that the audit is restricted to a clearly defined aspect of practice. Often, a simple tally chart collected by pen and paper is sufficient for the purposes of clinical audit.

The time over which the data are collected should be as short as is commensurate with collecting sufficient information to get a picture of what is happening. For example, the agreement may be to collect information on the next 100 consecutively attending patients. Alternatively, data could be collected for all patients over two weeks. Unlike in research studies, there is no need for a 'power calculation' to determine the required numbers.

4 Data analysis and reflection on results

Data analysis is usually restricted to simple counts and frequency analysis. There is no need for the application of statistical tests or calculation of probability values in clinical audits. The purpose of the analysis is to determine whether current practice meets the minimum standard agreed.

5 Agree and implement change

If the minimum standard is not being met, then it is necessary to agree and implement change to achieve it. Managing change is one of the greatest challenges that managers face. If changes are required, then there needs to be agreement on what changes are necessary, who will be responsible for making the changes, when this will occur and how. Staff can be reluctant to change, and it is important that they understand the reason for change and are provided with the necessary skills and resources to make change possible.

6 Monitor progress by repeating the cycle

What makes clinical audit a cyclical process is the necessity to repeat the audit sometime after the changes have been implemented to see whether they have had the desired effect and whether the minimum standard is now being achieved.

Features of a good clinical audit project

The features of a good clinical audit project are described in Table 49.2.

Practical aspects of clinical audit

The practical aspects that can limit the implementation of clinical audits are shown in Table 49.3.

Donabedian's triad

Donabedian described three elements of approaching healthcare quality. Clinical audits can be considered under these three headings:
- **Structure:** Looks at the amount and nature of staff, and facilities.
- **Process:** Looks at what is actually done to patients.
- **Outcome:** Looks at the results of treatment.

Peer review

Peer review is a quality assurance mechanism that operates alongside clinical audits. Peer review is less structured and less formal than clinical audit. In peer review, practitioners gather to discuss a clinical topic of mutual interest, often sharing details of clinical cases or problems. The theory is that by sharing ideas, solutions and standards will emerge by mutual consensus, and participants will learn from each other.

The difference between clinical audit and research

It is very important to appreciate the difference between clinical audit and clinical research.
- **Clinical research** is about extending the body of knowledge of best practices.
- **Clinical audit** is about measuring whether best practice is being applied.

50 Regulatory bodies and patient complaints

Table 50.1 The functions of the General Dental Council

Maintain the Dental Register

The GDC maintains registers of all dental professionals. This comprises registers of dentists and dental care professionals. The GDC also maintains a list of 13 dental specialties, which sets out who has undertaken additional training and is qualified as a Specialist. The registers are available online (www.gdc.org) and are searchable by anyone.

Investigate concerns and complaints about dental professionals

Through a *Fitness to Practice Committee*, the GDC investigates concerns about dental professionals. These may be on the grounds of *health; conduct* including convictions, cautions and *performance*.

Investigation can lead to a number of outcomes for the dental professional concerned:

• Being struck off the Dental Register so that they can no longer practise as a dental professional
• Suspension for a set period of time
• Being set conditions that restrict their practice
• A reprimand (a statement of disapproval)
• A finding of no case to answer.

Set and maintain educational standards

The GDC has defined the educational requirements for educational courses that qualify dentists and dental care professionals to enter the Dental Register or Specialists Lists. The GDC undertakes a series of inspections of dental schools and educational providers to ensure that the courses provided and the assessment of students undertaking these courses are of a minimum standard.

Continuing professional development

The GDC sets the requirements and maintains the record of continuing professional development for all dental professionals.

Overseas Registration Examination (ORE)

This examination, designed for dentists who have qualified outside the European Economic Area (EEA), is overseen by the GDC, and successful completion allows dentists to practise unsupervised in the UK.

Provision of information to patients

The GDC occasionally issues information for the public on topics of current interest, e.g. tooth whitening or travelling abroad for dental treatment.

Table 50.2 The fundamental standards of care expected by the Care Quality Commission

Standard	Patient Expectations that need to be satisfied
Person-centred care	You must have care or treatment that is tailored to you and meets your needs and preferences.
Dignity and respect	You must be treated with dignity and respect at all times while you're receiving care and treatment.
Consent	You (or anybody legally acting on your behalf) must consent before any care or treatment is given to you.
Safety	You must not be given unsafe care or treatment or be put at risk of harm that could be avoided.
Safeguarding from abuse	You must not suffer any form of abuse or improper treatment while receiving care.
Premises and equipment	The places where you receive care and treatment and the equipment used must be clean, suitable and looked after properly.
Complaints	You must be able to complain about your care and treatment.
Good governance	The provider of your care must have plans that ensure they can meet these standards.
Staffing	The provider of your care must have enough suitably qualified, competent and experienced staff to ensure they can meet these standards.
Fit and proper staff	The provider of your care must only employ people who can provide care and treatment appropriate to their role. They must have strong recruitment procedures in place and carry out relevant checks such as on applicants' criminal records and work history.
Duty of candour	The provider of your care must be open and transparent with you about your care and treatment.
Display of ratings	The provider of your care must display their CQC rating in a place where you can see it.

Dental Public Health at a Glance, Second Edition. Ivor G. Chestnutt.
© 2024 John Wiley & Sons Ltd. Published 2024 by John Wiley & Sons Ltd.

The regulation of dentistry

Dentistry is a profession regulated by statute, Section 38 of the Dentists Act 1984. It is, therefore, illegal for an individual to practise dentistry if they are not appropriately qualified and registered with the General Dental Council. The illegal practice of dentistry can lead to a criminal conviction and fine.

General Dental Council

The General Dental Council (GDC) is responsible for regulating the dental profession in the United Kingdom. Its functions are set out by Parliament, although it operates independently of both the government and the National Health Service. All dental professionals, irrespective of which sphere of dentistry they practise in, must be registered with the GDC and pay an annual fee to remain on the register.

The Council comprises six appointed registrants and six appointed lay members. It is the responsibility of the Council to ensure that the core responsibility of protecting patients is fulfilled.

The GDC describes its main functions as protecting patients and regulating the dental profession. This is achieved as set out in Table 50.1.

The nine professional principles

The GDC has set out nine principles to which all registrants and dental students must adhere:
* Put patients' interests first.
* Communicate effectively with patients
* Obtain valid consent
* Maintain and protect patients' information
* Have a clear and effective complaints procedure
* Work with colleagues in a way that is in patients' best interests
* Maintain, develop and work within your professional knowledge and skills
* Raise concerns if patients are at risk
* Make sure your personal behaviour maintains patients' confidence in you and the dental profession.

These standards are described in detail in a GDC publication, Standards for the Dental Team (www.gdc.org.uk). Failure to adhere to these standards can result in referral to the GDC and investigation under its 'fitness to practise' procedures.

The Care Quality Commission (CQC)

The Care Quality Commission (CQC) is the independent regulator of health and social care in England. All dental providers in England must register with the CQC. Its purpose is to ensure that health and social care services provide people with safe, effective, compassionate, high-quality care and to encourage care services to improve. The CQC has described what patients can expect from healthcare providers (Table 50.2).

The role of the CQC is to inspect and regulate services to ensure they meet fundamental standards of quality and safety. It publishes the results of inspections, which are available for anyone to read on the CQC website. Dentists must pay an annual fee to remain registered with the CQC.

Following an inspection of a dental practice, the CQC will report on compliance in the following areas:
* Treating people with respect and involving them in their care
* Providing care, treatment and support that meet people's needs
* Caring for people safely and protecting them from harm
* Staffing
* Quality and suitability of management.

Failure to meet the required standard may result in the issue of an enforcement notice.

Health Inspectorate Wales (HIW) performs a similar function to the CGC in Wales, as does **Healthcare Improvement Scotland (HIS)** in Scotland.

Patient complaints

The most common causes of complaints in dental practice are failure in communication, disputes over monetary charges and failure of clinical treatment.

Effective and efficient management of patients' concerns and complaints is important, as resolution at an early stage may prevent the scenarios outlined in Table 48.1. It is always preferable that a patient's complaint or concern be resolved informally. However, if the patient wishes to complain formally, the options available depend on whether their treatment was carried out under the National Health Service or Independently.

The NHS complaints process

This has two stages:
* **Stage 1**: Local resolution. Here, the patient makes a formal complaint to the dentist or the commissioner of the service. If the patient remains unsatisfied with the solution offered, then Stage 2 may be invoked.
* **Stage 2**: Complaint to the Parliamentary and Health Service Ombudsman. This stage is reserved for more serious complaints that cannot be resolved by local resolution.

Complaints about private dental care

The Dental Complaints Service comprises a team of trained advisers whose aim is to help private dental patients and dental professionals settle complaints about private dental care fairly and efficiently.

Patients may also complain directly to the General Dental Council. It is suggested that patients are more willing to complain about the care they receive from their dentist than has been the case in the past.

Responding to a complaint

A dentist or dental care professional who receives a formal complaint should seek advice from their indemnity organisation on resolving the patient's complaint. Dental practices should have an in-house complaints procedure and a dedicated complaints manager.

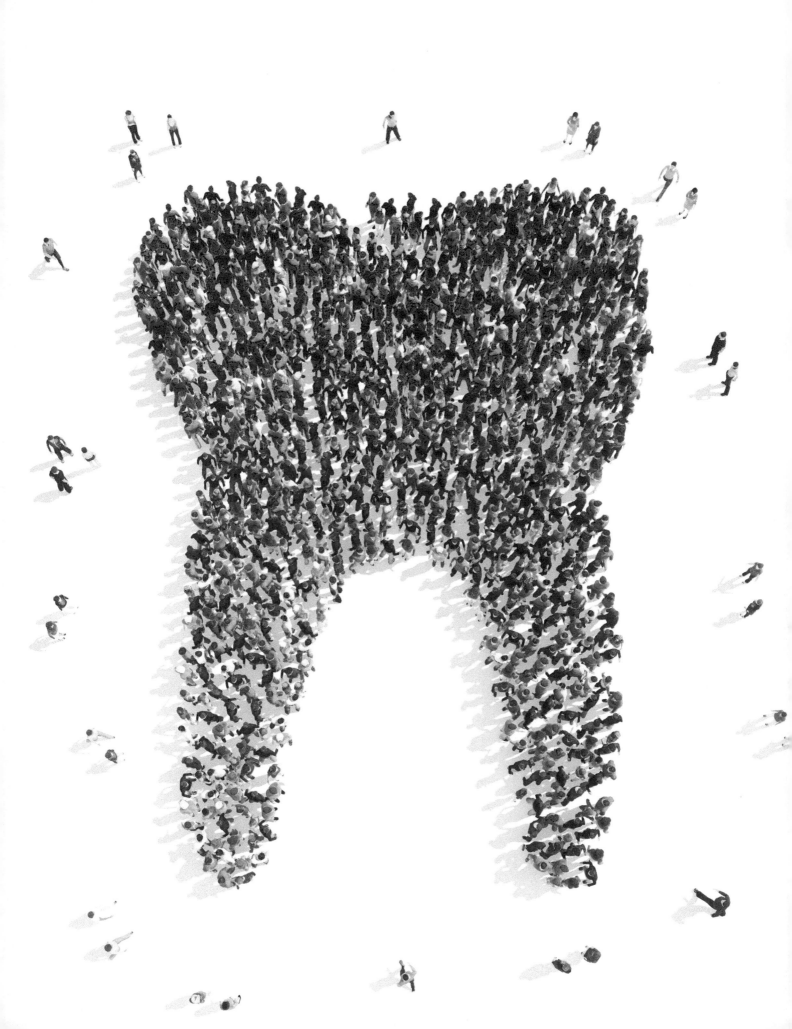

A career in dental public health

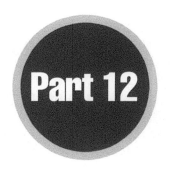

Part 12

Chapters

51 A career in dental public health

A career in dental public health

It is to be hoped that by this stage, readers of this book will realise that an appreciation of oral health and dental services from a population perspective is a necessary skill for all dental professionals. The promotion of oral health at the chairside on an individual basis and advocacy for oral health on a general level are core components of the role of all members of the dental team.

Those working in Community Dental Services will be required to fulfil key elements of the dental public health function, such as participation in epidemiological surveys and data collection and the organisation and delivery of national or regional oral health improvement programmes.

Around the world, dental public health professionals have a key role to play in organising the development of dental services and advocating for oral health.

Dental public health training

In the United Kingdom, dental public health is recognised as a specialty by the General Dental Council (GDC). In order to claim specialist status, a dentist must have undergone a formal programme of training, have been awarded a Certificate of Completion of Specialist Training (CCST) by the Dental Postgraduate Deanery and be on the Specialist List of the GDC.

The formal dental public health training programme in the UK lasts four years. One year will be spent undertaking a Master's in (Dental) Public Health. A defined curriculum for dental public health specialist training has been devised by the GDC and is available on its website. Training programmes are organised by and run under the auspices of the Dental Postgraduate Deanery. The Specialist Advisory Committee in Dental Public Health of the Royal College of Surgeons of England provides quality assurance of the training programmes. However, the responsibility for approval lies with the Dental Postgraduate Dean.

Upon completing the training programme, trainees take the Intercollegiate Specialty Fellowship Examination (ISFE) in Dental Public Health. Successful completion of this examination, together with successful completion of the training programme, enables the trainee to be awarded a CCST and thus to apply for admission to the GDC Specialist List.

Registration on the GDC Specialist List is a necessary precondition of appointment to a consultant in dental public health post in the National Health Service.

Specialists/consultants in dental public health work in two main roles. The majority are employed by the National Health Service. They work with key stakeholders from a broad range of backgrounds on the improvement of oral health and delivery of dental services. The alternative role for specialists/consultants in dental public health is in academia. Here, they are employed by a university, and the main focus of their role is research and teaching.

Anyone interested in a career in dental public health should discuss this with their local consultant in dental public health or with the Dental Postgraduate Deanery. Alternatively, the Chairperson of the Specialist Advisory Committee in Dental Public Health can be contacted via the Royal College of Surgeons of England.

Dental Public Health at a Glance, Second Edition. Ivor G. Chestnutt.
© 2024 John Wiley & Sons Ltd. Published 2024 by John Wiley & Sons Ltd.

References and selected useful resources and further reading

References

Bradshaw, J. (1972) Taxonomy of social need. In G. McLachlan (ed), *Problems and Progress in Medical Care: Essays on Current Research*, 7th series (pp. 71–82). London: Oxford University Press.

Buchanan, H., Newton, J.T., Baker, S.R., and Asimakopoulou K. (2021) Adopting the COM-B model and TDF framework in oral and dental research: a narrative review. *Community Dentistry and Oral Epidemiology*, 49: 385–393.

Burden, D.J., Pine, C.M., and Burnside, G. (2001) Modified IOTN: an orthodontic treatment need index for use in oral health surveys. *Community Dentistry and Oral Epidemiology*, 29: 220–5.

Cane, J., O'Connor, D., and Michie, S. (2012) Validation of the theoretical domains framework for use in behaviour change and implementation research. *Implementation Science*, 7: 37.

Dahlgren, G. and Whitehead, M. (1991) *Policies and Strategies to Promote Social Equity in Health*. Stockholm: Institute for Futures Studies.

General Dental Council (2013) *Scope of Practice*. https://www.gdc-uk.org/docs/default-source/scope-of-practice/scope-of-practice.pdf

General Dental Council (2022) *Registration Statistical Report*. https://www.gdc-uk.org/docs/default-source/annual-reports/gdc_registration-statistical-report-22-23-v3_a.pdf

Greene, J.C. and Vermillion, J.R. (1960) Oral hygiene index: a method for classifying oral hygiene status. *Journal of the American Dental Association*, 61: 172–179.

Hayden, C, Bowler, J.O., Chambers, S. et al. (2013) Obesity and dental caries in children: a systematic review and meta-analysis. *Community Dentistry and Oral Epidemiology*, 41: 289–308.

Health and Social Care Information Centre (2011) *1: Oral Health and Function – A Report from the Adult Dental Health Survey 2009*. https://doc.ukdataservice.ac.uk/doc/6884/mrdoc/pdf/6884theme1_oral_health_and_function.pdf

Löe, H. (1967) The gingival index, the plaque index and the retention index systems. *Journal of Periodontology*, 38: S610–S616.

Mariño, R., Ravisankar, G., and Zaror, C. (2020) Quality appraisal of economic evaluations done on oral health preventive programs – a systematic review. *Journal Public Health Dentistry*, 80: 194–207.

Marshman, Z., Ainsworth, H., Chestnutt, I.G. et al. (2019). Brushing RemInder 4 Good oral HealTh (BRIGHT) trial: does an SMS behaviour change programme with a classroom-based session improve the oral health of young people living in deprived areas? A study protocol of a randomised controlled trial. *Trials*, 20. https://doi.org/10.1186/s13063-019-3538-6.

NHS Digital (2015) *Child Dental Health Survey 2013, England Wales and Northern Ireland – NHS Digital*. https://digital.nhs.uk/data-and-information/publications/statistical/children-s-dental-health-survey/child-dental-health-survey-2013-england-wales-and-northern-ireland

NHS England Digital Analytical Team (2014) https://www.england.nhs.uk/wp-content/uploads/2014/02/dental-info-pack.pdf

Office for National Statistics (2018) *Smoking Inequalities in England, 2016*. https://www.ons.gov.uk/peoplepopulationandcommunity/healthandsocialcare/drugusealcoholandsmoking/adhocs/008181smokinginequalitiesinengland2016

Prochaska, J.O. and DiClemente, C.C. (1982) Transtheoretical therapy: Toward a more integrative model of change. *Psychotherapy: Theory, Research & Practice*, 19: 276–288.

Public Health England (2018) *Carbon Modelling within Dentistry: Towards a Sustainable Future*. https://assets.publishing.service.gov.uk/media/5b461fa2e5274a37893e3928/Carbon_modelling_within_dentistry.pdf

Rosenstock, I.M., Strecher, V.J., Marshall, H., and Becker, H. (1988) Social learning theory and the health belief model. *Health Education Quarterly*, 15: 175–183.

Ruiz, B., Broadbent, J.M., Thomson, W.M. et al. (2023) Differential unmet needs and experience of restorative dental care in trajectories of dental caries experience: a birth cohort study. *Caries Ressearch*, 57: 524–535.

Scally, G and Donaldson, L.J. (1998) Clinical governance and the drive for quality improvement in the new NHS in England. *British Medical Journal*, 317: 61–65.

Sheiham, A. and Watt, R. (2001) The Common Risk Factor Approach: a rational basis for promoting oral health. *Community Dentistry and Oral Epidemiology*, 28: 399–406.

Siemieniuk, R. and Guyatt, G. (2023) *What is GRADE?* https://bestpractice.bmj.com/info/toolkit/learn-ebm/what-is-grade/

Silness, J. and Löe, H. (1964) Periodontal disease in pregnancy. II. Correlation between oral hygiene and periodontal condition. *Acta Odontologica Scandiniavia*, 22: 121–135.

Slade, G. (1997) Derivation and validation of a short-form oral health impact profile. *Community Dentistry and Oral Epidemiology*, 25(4): 284–290. https://doi.org/10.1111/j.1600-0528.1997.tb00941.x. This paper provides the original description of the OHIP-14 questionnaire.

Smoke-free and Smiling (2014) *Guidance on Helping Dental Patients to Quit Smoking*. https://www.gov.uk/government/publications/smokefree-and-smiling

UK Government Office for Health Improvement and Disparities (2022) *Nicotine Vaping in England: 2022 Evidence Update*. https://www.gov.uk/government/publications/nicotine-vaping-in-england-2022-evidence-update

Wilson, J.M.G. and Junger, G. (1968) The principles and practice of screening for disease. *Public Health Papers*, 34. Geneva: World Health Organization. http://apps.who.int/iris/bitstream/10665/37650/1/WHO_PHP_34.pdf

World Health Organisation (2015a) *Fact Sheet: Waterpipe Tobacco Smoking and Health*. https://www.who.int/publications/i/item/fact-sheet-waterpipe-tobacco-smoking-and-health

World Health Organisation (2015b) *Guideline: Sugars Intake for Adults and Children*. http://www.who.int/nutrition/publications/guidelines/sugars_intake/en/

World Health Organisation (2021) *WHO Global Report on Trends in Prevalence of Tobacco Use 2000–2025, Third Edition*. https://www.who.int/publications/i/item/9789240039322

World Health Organisation (2022) *Global Oral Health Status Report: Towards Universal Health Coverage for Oral Health by 2030*. https://www.who.int/publications/i/item/9789240061484

World Health Organisation (2023) *Climate Change and Health*. https://www.who.int/teams/environment-climate-change-and-health/climate-change-and-health

World Health Organisation (2015) Guideline: Sugars Intake for Adults and Children. Recommended Sugar Intakes. https://www.who.int/publications/i/item/9789241549028

World Health Organisation Global Oral Health Data Portal (2015) This site gives access to the WHO's global database – it can be used to determine oral disease prevalence (where available) in countries around the world. https://www.who.int/data/gho/data/themes/oral-health-data-portal

Yang, Z., Sun, P., Dahlstrom, K.R. et al. (2023) Joint effect of human papillomavirus exposure, smoking and alcohol on risk of oral squamous cell carcinoma. *BMC Cancer*, 23: 457.

Selected useful resources and further reading

British Association for the Study of Community Dentistry. BASCD is the UK's professional association for the science, philosophy and practice of promoting the oral health of populations and groups in society. www.bascd.org/

British Dental Association (BDA) is the professional association and trade union for dentists in the United Kingdom and was founded in 1880. www.bda.org/

British Fluoridation Society. The BFS aims to encourage fluoridation of the water supply. http://www.bfsweb.org

Cancer Research UK. Contains a useful database on oral cancer. www.cancerresearchuk.org/

Care Quality Commission, www.cqc.org.uk/ Describes the functions of the CQC as they relate to dentistry and reports of the inspection of dental practices in England.

Cochrane Library. A repository of systematic reviews. http://www.cochranelibrary.com/

Faculty of Public Health The professional organization in the United Kingdom for generic public health. www.fph.org.uk/

General Dental Council. The body is responsible for the registration of dental professionals and oversight of standards and dental education. https://www.gdc-uk.org/

Health Education England. Provides information about Specialty training in Dental Public Health in England. https://dental.hee.nhs.uk/dental-trainee-recruitment/dental-specialty-training/dental-public-health/overview-of-dental-public-health/dental-public-health-overview

Health Education and Improvement Wales. Responsible for postgraduate dental training in Wales, including specialty training in Dental Public Health. https://heiw.nhs.wales/

NHS Education for Scotland. Responsible for postgraduate education, including specialty training in dental public health in Scotland. https://www.nes.scot.nhs.uk/

NHS Digital, Adult Dental Health Survey 2009 - Summary report and thematic series. This site holds the results of the 2009 adult dental health survey https://digital.nhs.uk/data-and-information/publications/statistical/adult-dental-health-survey/adult-dental-health-survey-2009-summary-report-and-thematic-series

NHS England. Dentistry Leading the change for oral health. Site of the Chief Dental Officer for England. https://www.england.nhs.uk/primary-care/dentistry/leading-the-change/

National Institute for Health and Care Excellence. NICE provides national guidance and advice to improve health and social care. www.nice.org.uk

Office for National Statistics. This site holds data on many aspects of life in the United Kingdom, population data, data from various national surveys and decennial censuses. https://www.ons.gov.uk/

Royal College of Surgeons of Edinburgh, www.rcsed.ac.uk/

Royal College of Surgeons of England, www.rcseng.ac.uk/ This college hosts the Specialty Advisory Committee on Dental Public Health. It also holds the Diploma in Dental Public Health Examinations.

Royal College of Physicians and Surgeons of Glasgow, www.rcpsg.ac.uk/ This College hosts the Intercollegiate Specialty Examination in Dental Public Health on behalf of all four Royal Colleges.

Royal College of Surgeons in Ireland, www.rcsi.ie/

Scottish Dental. A repository of information from NHS Scotland about dentistry in Scotland. https://www.scottishdental.org/

Scottish National Dental Inspection Programme. Contains the results of dental epidemiological surveys in Scotland. https://ndip.scottishdental.org/

United Kingdom Health Security Agency. Describes the health protection function of the NHS. https://www.gov.uk/government/organisations/uk-health-security-agency

Welsh Oral Health Information Unit. This site is the repository for oral health surveys in Wales. https://www.cardiff.ac.uk/research/explore/research-units-old/welsh-oral-health-information-unit

Index

acculturation, 104
acquired immune deficiency syndrome (AIDS), 23
acute necrotising gingivitis, 23
adult dental health survey, 45
advertisements, 49
advocacy, 49
alcohol, 16, 31, 48, 82, 83
    brief intervention, 83
    minimum unit price, 83
    misuse, 83
    recommended safe levels of consumption, 82
    units, 82
alcoholism, 83
animal studies, 69
antiretroviral therapy 23
arginine, 61
armed forces dentistry, 88
aspartame, 71
assessment, 2
Assessment of Clinical Oral Risks and Needs (ACORN), 55
association, 26
assurance, 2

bands-of dental care, 101, 113
barriers to dental care, 102
Basic Periodontal Examination (BPE), 10
behaviour change, 50
    theories, 50
    wheel, 52
betel quid, 16, 77
bias, 27
    publication, 38
    recall, 31, 33
    selection, 33
bidi, 77
binge drinking, 83
biofilm, 59
biological plausibility, 27
blended dental contract, 101
blind, 35
    single, 35
    triple, 35
Bradford-Hill criteria, 27
breastfeeding, 69
brief intervention, 83
BRIGHT Clinical Trial, 35
British Association for the Study of Community Dentistry (BASCD), 13, 29, 65
British Fluoridation Society, 62
British Orthodontic Society, 41
British Society for Periodontology, 41
Bullying, 49

BUPA, 101
bupropion, 79

calculus, 61
calibration, 35
cancer, 48
candida (thrush), 23
cannabis, 77
Capability Opportunity Motivation-Behaviour Model, 53
capitation, 101, 113
carbon footprint, 111
cardiovascular disease, 48, 65
Care Quality Commission (CQC), 97, 120
case-control study, 27, 30
case report, 28
cause, 27, 29
Childsmile, 65
CINHAL, 39
citation chaning, 39
climate change, 111
clinical audit, 117, 118
    criteria, 119
    cycle, 119
    outcome, 119
    process, 119
    standards, 119
    structure, 119
clinical dental technician, 107
clinical effectiveness, 116
clinical governance, 116
clinical guideline, 41
    adherence, 41
    certainty of the evidence, 41
clinical research, 119
Cochrane Collaboration, 38, 40
Cochrane Library, 41
Cochrane Professor Archie, 40
cohort study, 27, 32
College of General Dentistry, 119
commercial determinants of health, 71
commissioning NHS dental services, 98
commom risk factor approach, 48
Community Dental Service, 98
community network, 5
Community Periodontal Index of Treatment Need (CPITN), 10, 15
complaints, 120, 121
    Dental Complaints Service, 121
    responding to a complaint, 121
complex intervention, 49
confounding, 27, 29
CONSORT-statement, 35
continuing professional development, 117

Dental Public Health at a Glance, Second Edition. Ivor G. Chestnutt.
© 2024 John Wiley & Sons Ltd. Published 2024 by John Wiley & Sons Ltd.